QUIZ TIME

SCIENCE & TECHNOLOGY

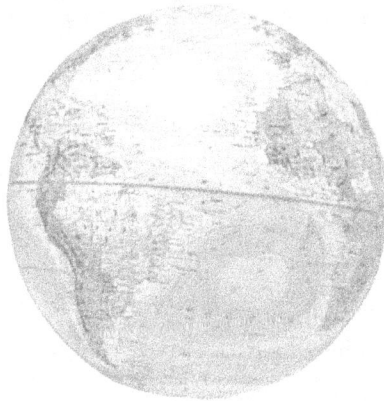

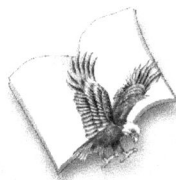

V&S PUBLISHERS

Published by:

V&S PUBLISHERS

F-2/16, Ansari road, Daryaganj, New Delhi-110002
☎ 23240026, 23240027 • *Fax:* 011-23240028
Email: info@vspublishers.com • *Website:* www.vspublishers.com

Regional Office : Hyderabad

5-1-707/1, Brij Bhawan (Beside Central Bank of India Lane)
Bank Street, Koti, Hyderabad - 500 095
☎ 040-24737290
E-mail: vspublishershyd@gmail.com

Branch Office : Mumbai

Jaywant Industrial Estate, 1st Floor–108, Tardeo Road
Opposite Sobo Central Mall, Mumbai – 400 034
☎ 022-23510736
E-mail: vspublishersmum@gmail.com

Follow us on:

© **Copyright:** *V&S PUBLISHERS*
Edition 2018

Publisher's Note

As per its name, **V&S Publishers** is known for books of **Value** and **Substance** pertaining to every possible subject of general interest, such as: Personality Development, Health and Nutrition, Management Studies, Children Encyclopaedia, Storybooks, Science books for school students, Dictionaries on Physics, Chemistry Biology, Economics, Mathematics, etc. **Quiz Time** is a decade-old series containing best-sellers like on Quizzing. This book, *Quiz Time-Science & Technology* is yet answer addition to this series.

The book includes an exclusive collection of more than **400 informative, interesting and brain teasing questions** along with their **answers** on:

❖ Physical and Life Sciences
❖ Information Technology
❖ Mathematics
❖ Environment
❖ Cinema

The book aims to educate and enlighten all its readers, particularly the student section and the ones trying to crack various competitive examinations.

Hope the book helps to enhance your General Knowledge and serves its purpose well!

Contents

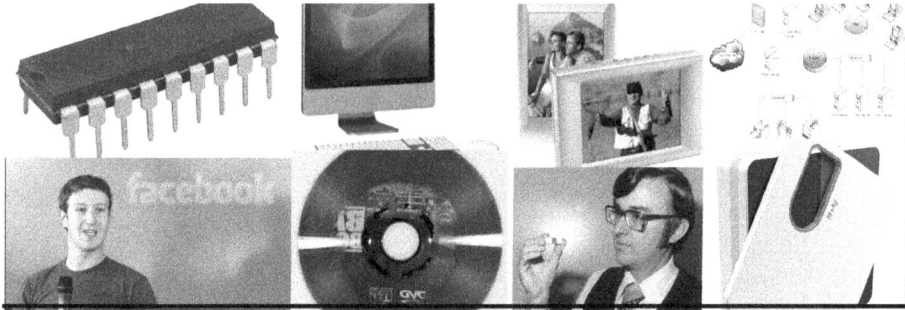

SCIENCE

&

LIVING SCIENCE

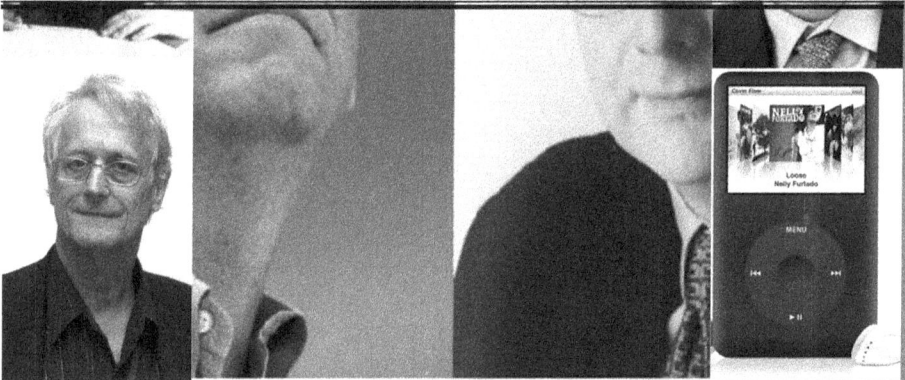

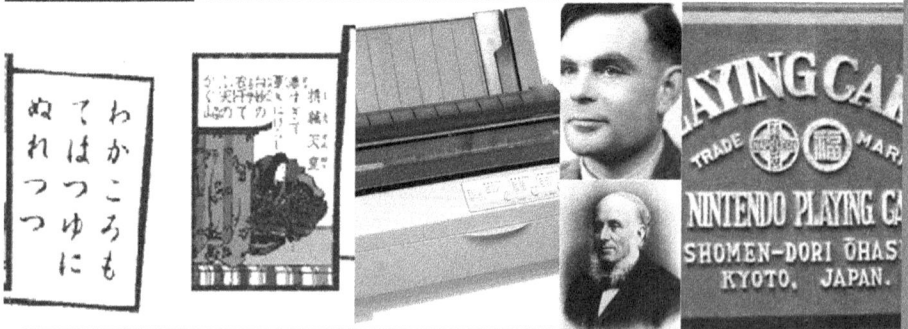

Q-1. What is made up of a variety of materials such as Carbon and inhibits the flow of current?

Ans. Resistor

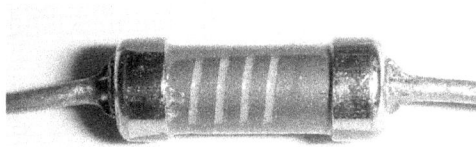

Carbon resistor

Q-2. Global warming is due to increased production of which gas?

Ans. Carbon dioxide

Q-3. Which acid is present in lemon?

Ans. Citric acid

Q-4. Brass is an alloy of which two metals?

Ans. Copper and Zinc

Q-5. Which is the hardest natural substance found in the world?

Ans. Diamond

Q-6. Which substance helps in removing the permanent hardness of the water?

Ans. Sodium Carbonate

Q-7. Which is the most commonly used bleaching agent?

Ans. Chlorine

Q-8. Which gas is used in cigarette lighter?

Ans. Butane

Q-9. What is the common name of Sodium Bicarbonate?

Ans. Baking Soda

Q-10. What are the atoms of the same element having the same atomic numbers but different atomic weights called?

Ans. Isotopes

Q-11. What is the main constituent of soap?

Ans. Sodium Hydroxide

Q-12. Name a fertilizer that contains maximum amount of Nitrogen.

Ans. Urea

Q-13. Which compound is called Oil of Wintergreen?

Ans. Methyl Salicylate

Q-14. What is alum?

Ans. Potassium Aluminium Silicate

Q-15. Name an alloy of copper, antimony and tin.

Ans. Babbitt metal

Q-16. Famous New Zealand scientist Ernest Rutherford was awarded a Nobel Prize in which field?

Ans. Chemistry

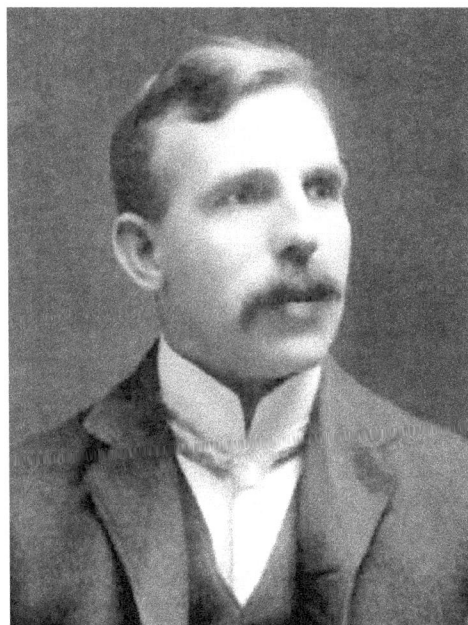

Ernest Rutherford

Q-17. What is the name given to substances that are initially involved in a chemical reaction?

Ans. Reactants

Q-18. What is the fourth most abundant element in the universe in terms of mass?

Ans. Carbon

Q-19. Is sodium hydroxide (NaOH) an acid or base?

Ans. Base

Q-20. At room temperature what is the only metal that is in liquid form?

Ans. Mercury

Q-21. What is the centre of an atom called?

Ans. Nucleus

Q-22. K is the chemical symbol for which element?

Ans. Potassium

Q-23. A nuclear reaction where the nucleus of an atom splits into smaller parts is known as nuclear fission or nuclear fusion?

Ans. Nuclear Fission

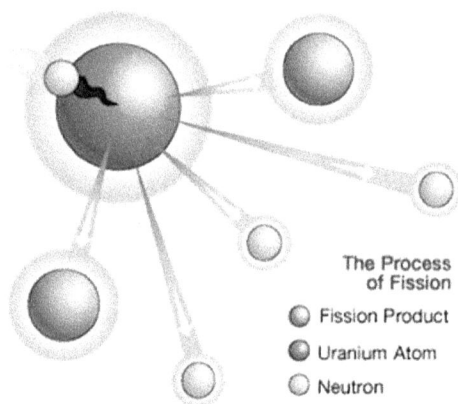

The Process of Fission

◯ Fission Product
◯ Uranium Atom
◯ Neutron

Nuclear fission reaction

Q-24. What is the chemical symbol for gold?

Ans. Au

Q-25. What orbits the nucleus of an atom?

Ans. Electrons

Q-26. H_2O is liquid, but what is H_2S?

Ans. Gas

Q-27. Which element on adding to natural rubber makes it less sticky in hot weather and less hard in cold weather?

Ans. Sulphur

Q-28. What is a raincoat made up of?

Ans. Polychloroethene

Q-29. Which element can easily form chains?

Ans. Carbon

Q-30. Which element is used as an antichlor?

Ans. SO_2

Q-31. Which catalyst used in the manufacture of ammonia from nitrogen and hydrogen?

Ans. Iron

Q-32. Which element can be toxic to plants growing in soils that are high in acidity?

Ans. Aluminum

Q-33. Glass is made out of what?

Ans. Sand

Q-34. Which drug is present in cola drinks?

Ans. Caffeine

Q-35. Which drug is present in tobacco?

Ans. Nicotine

Q-36. Which element is present in the least amount in a living body?

Ans. Manganese

Q-37. What is the most common natural source for sulphur?

Ans. Volcanic region

Q-38. Which when dissolved in water gives hissing sound?

Ans. Limestone

Q-39. Which gas is also called Stranger Gas?

Ans. Xenon

Q-40. What are Rubies and Sapphires chemically known as?

Ans. Aluminium Oxides

Q-41. Which substance is used as a mordant in dying and tanning industry?

Ans. Magnesium Sulphate

Q-42. Mixture of which pairs of gases is the cause of occurrence of most of the explosion in mines?

Ans. Methane and air

Q-43. Which common device works on the basis of the principle of mutual induction?

Ans. Transformer

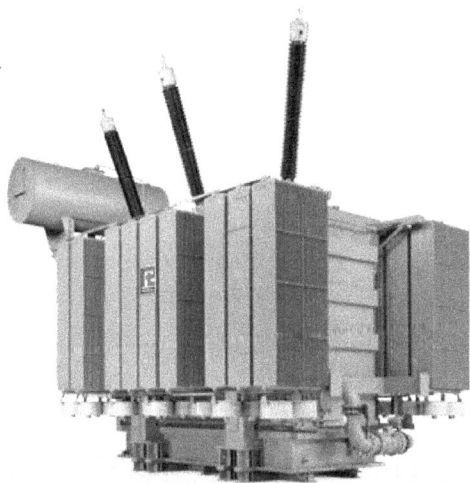

Transformer

Q-44. DC current can be controlled by which component?

Ans. Resistor

Q-45. Mesons are found in _____.

Ans. Cosmic rays

Q-46. Which substance is used as a moderator in nuclear reactor?

Ans. Graphite

Q-47. In an atomic nucleus, neutrons and protons are held together by _____.

Ans. Exchange forces

Q-48. Due to what Television signal cannot be received generally beyond a particular distance.

Ans. Curvature of earth

Q-49. What is the main component of biogas and natural gas?

Ans. Methane

Q-50. Aviation fuel for Jet aeroplanes consists of purified _____.

Ans. Kerosene

Q-51. Who invented Bakelite?

Ans. Leo Hendrik Baekeland

Q-52. Cyrogenic engines find application in _____.

Ans. Rocket technology

Q-53. What is the main constituent of coal gas?

Ans. Methane

Q-54. A red object when seen through a thick blue glass appears of which colour?

Ans. Black

Q-55. On what conservation laws does a rocket work?

Ans. Angular momentum

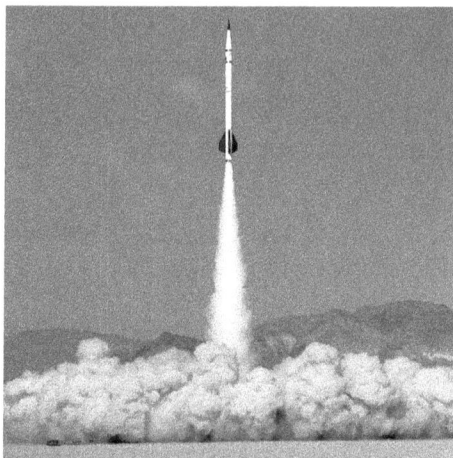

Rocket launching

Q-56. Where is the Central Arid Zone Research Institute (CAZRI) located?

Ans. Jodhpur

Q-57. Which rare element would you associate with Marie and Pierre Curie?

Ans. Radium

Q-58. What process used to separate the different components of oil?

Ans. Fractional Distillation

TRIVIA

The process Fractional Distillation is based on the fact that the different components of oil have different boiling points. In this process, oil is heated in a furnace to 400 degree Celsius (752 F) and it vapourises. The vapours are introduced into a tall fractionating column. There the component vapours condense one by one at different heights. The vapours with lower boiling points condense at the top and those with higher boiling points condense near the bottom. The various fractions are then collected from the column. Some of them are – Petroleum gas, gasoline, kerosene, diesel, fuel oil, lubricating oil, wax and asphalt.

Q-59. Which variety of coal contains the highest percentage of carbon?

Ans. Anthracite

Q-60. If you wanted to lighten your hair at home, what is the active ingredient used the dye preparation that will lighten your hair?

Ans. Hydrogen Perioxide

Q-61. Aspirin can be found in many household medicine cabinets. But what is it chemically?

Ans. Acetylsalicylic acid

Q-62. "Antifreeze" is used in car radiators to stop the liquid that cools the engine from freezing when it gets cold outside. Water is one component of antifreeze; what is the other main component?

Ans. Ethylene glycol

Q-63. What is dry ice?

Ans. Solid Carbon Dioxide

TRIVIA

"Dry ice" is solid carbon dioxide (CO_2). Carbon dioxide freezes at -78.5 degrees Centigrade. When dry ice "melts" it undergoes a process called sublimation. This means that it is converted from a solid directly to a gas, bypassing the intermediate liquid stage. This is where the name "dry ice" comes from – when it melts, you never get any liquid (unlike water ice), hence it's "dry".

Q-64. What is the major component of the adhesive–woodworking glue also known as PVA glue?

Ans. Poly Vinyl Alcohol

Q-65. What is it in nail polish remover that does the polish removing?

Ans. Acetone

Q-66. What is the main component of household bleach?

Ans. Sodium hypochlorite

Q-67. Methylated spirits is a very common household chemical, but what is its main component?

Ans. Ethanol

Q-68. Which chemical compound occurs naturally in tea and coffee and is a popular additive to soft drinks?

Ans. Caffeine

Q-69. How many moons does Pluto have (found by year 2000)?

Ans. One

Q-70. Which planet orbits the sun at a speed of 110,000 kph?

Ans. Earth

Q-71. A meteorite struck Antarctica in 2004. It was 30 feet wide. How far away was the climate affected by this strike?

Ans. Other side of the planet

Q-72. In the 1990s, a spacecraft was designed to protect Earth from meteors, asteroids and comets. What was its name?

Ans. Clementine II

TRIVIA

Anything that might hit Earth is called a Near Earth Object.

Q-73. The most famous meteor shower is the Perseids. What is its other name?

Ans. Tears of Saint Lawrence

Q-74. What does Candela measure?

Ans. Luminous Intensity

Q-75. Which of the "rare" gases is most common in the atmosphere?

Ans. Xenon

Q-76. What type of storm has a central calm area, called the eye, which has winds spiraling inwardly?

Ans. Thunderstorm

Q-77. What is the pH of Acid rain?

Ans. 6

Q-78. Which two metals are mixed in manufacturing of stainless steel?

Ans. Chromium and iron

Q-79. How much body heat escapes from our body to cool off?

Ans. 80%

Q-80. What measurement unit microbiologists use when they want to measure something really small (like a bacterial cell)?

Ans. Micrometer

Q-81. What organelle is known as the 'brain' of the cell?

Ans. Nucleus

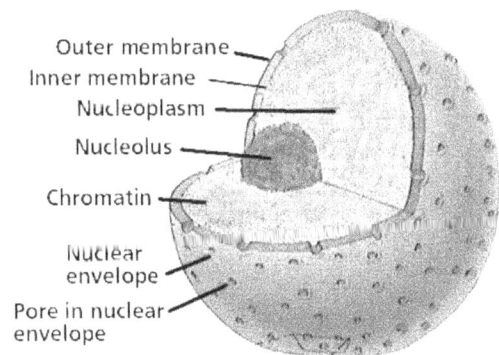

Outer membrane
Inner membrane
Nucleoplasm
Nucleolus
Chromatin
Nuclear envelope
Pore in nuclear envelope

Cell structure

Q-82. A _____ beam is one whose rays remain the same distance apart.

Ans. Parallel

Q-83. Materials through which light cannot pass are known as _____.

Ans. Opaque

Q-84. What are those bodies called which radiate light?

Ans. Luminous

Q-85. Most of the magnetic power appears to be concentrated at certain points of a magnet. These points are called _____.

Ans. Poles

Q-86. The law that "the physical and chemical properties of elements are periodic functions of their atomic weights" was given by whom?

Ans. Mendeleev

Q-87. Who gave the Law of Octaves?

Ans. John Newlands

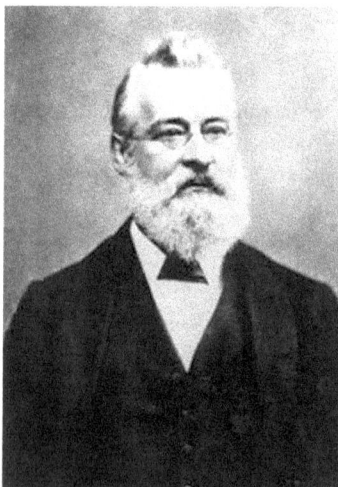

John Newlands

Q-88. With which metal does oxygen combine to form rust?

Ans. Iron

Q-89. Rocks that are rich in metals are known as _____.

Ans. Ores

Q-90. Which metal is often found in the pure state?

Ans. Gold

Q-91. Which gland is in the shape of pistol?

Ans. Pancreas

Q-92. Which organ produces bile juice?

Ans. Liver

TRIVIA

Liver produces around one litre of bile juice per day.

Q-93. Folic acid is also known as _____.

Ans. Vitamin M

Q-94. Which test is used to know colour blindness?

Ans. Ishihara

Q-95. Fear of water is known as _____.

Ans. Hydrophobia

Q-96. Aviophobia is fear of what?

Ans. Fear of flying

Q-97. Claustrophobia is fear of what?

Ans. Fear of confined spaces

TRIVIA

Paraskavedekatriaphobia or Paraskevidekatriaphobia or Friggatriskaidekaphobia is the fear of Friday the 13th.

Q-98. Which is the world's largest private international nature conservation organisation?

Ans. World Wide Fund for nature

Q-99. Which animal can look at two ways at the same time?

Ans. Chameleon

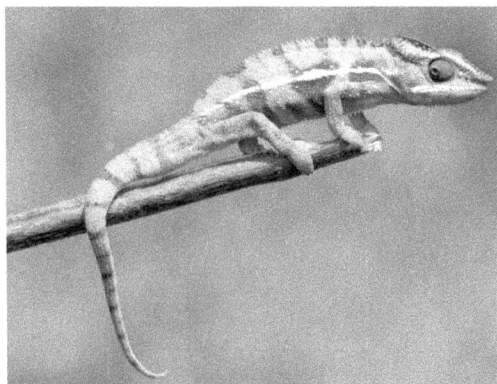

Chameleon

Q-100. Which Indian region is the only place in the world where the Asiatic Wild Ass is found?

Ans. Rann of Kachchh

Q-101. What is the gestation period of an African elephant?

Ans. 22 Months

Q-102. Which bird constructs the largest unit nest structure in the world?

Ans. Sociable Weaver

Q-103. Who wrote 'Origin of species'?

Ans. Charles Darwin

Q-104. Which animal is the main attraction in Assam's Kaziranga National Park?

Ans. The one-horned rhinoceros

Q-105. World Wildlife Fund was founded in which year?

Ans. 1961

Q-106. Who wrote the autobiographical book, My Life: My Trees?

Ans. Richard St. Barbe Baker

Q-107. On which day World Oceans Day falls on?

Ans. June 8

Q-108. Who discovered Penicillin?

Ans. Alexander Fleming

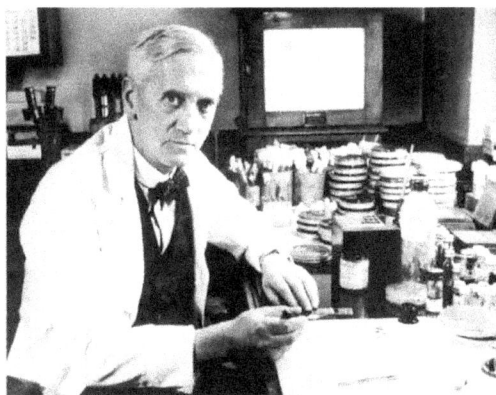

Alexander Fleming

Q-109. Who discovered treatment for rabies?

Ans. Louis Pasteur

Q-110. Who discovered chloroform?

Ans. Simpson and Harrison

Q-111. Who discovered anti-polio vaccine?

Ans. Jonas E. Salk

Q-112. Who discovered the cause of beri beri disease?

Ans. Eijkman

Q-113. The absence of cobalt in minute quantities in human body causes what?

Ans. Pernicious anaemia

Q-114. What is the full form of DNA?

Ans. Deoxyribonucleic Acid

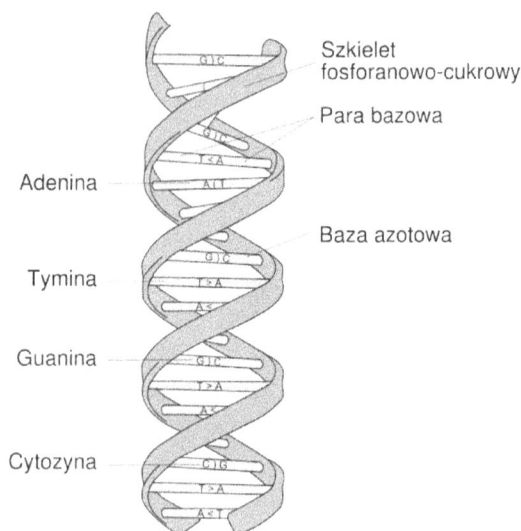

DNA structure

Q-115. Which is the free living bacterium that fixes nitrogen?

Ans. Azotobacter

Q-116. What is exobiology?

Ans. It is the study of life in outer space

Q-117. Which vitamin is abundant in citrus fruits?

Ans. Vitamin C

Q-118. Which gas in the atmosphere saves us from the ultra-violet rays of the sun?

Ans. Ozone

Q-119. What is the more common name for a polymer of amino acids?

Ans. Protein

Q-120. What is the study of flowers called?

Ans. Anthology

Q-121. The largest living animals belong to the group of _____.

Ans. Mammals

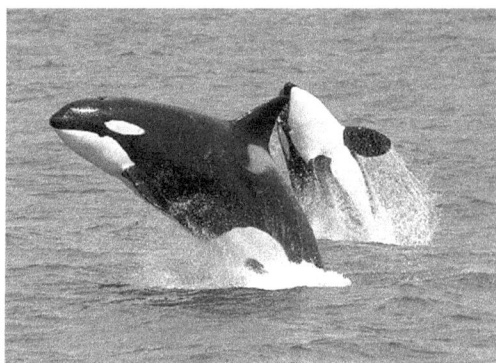

Whale

Q-122. _____ are made up of oxygen, carbon and hydrogen.

Ans. Carbohydrates

Q-123. There are twelve pairs of _____ nerves in the human body.

Ans. Cranial

Q-124. Which animal was used by Edward Jenner to prepare vaccine?

Ans. Calves

Q-125. What the rearing of silkworm is known as?

Ans. Sericulture

Q-126. Which vitamin is destroyed by cooking?

Ans. Vitamin C

Q-127. Which vitamin is responsible for anti-sterile activities?

Ans. Vitamin E

Q-128. The upper chambers of the heart are called _____.

Ans. Atria

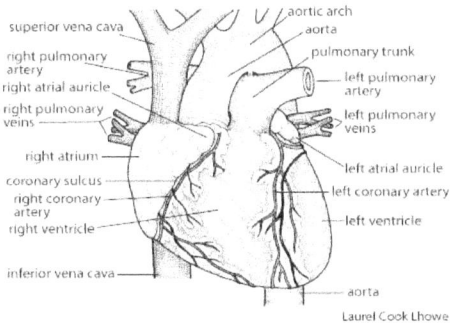

Heart structure

Q-129. Kwashiorkor is caused due to deficiency of what?

Ans. Protein

Q-130. What are known as the fundamental units of kidney?

Ans. Nephrons

Q-131. Which is the master gland in the endocrine orchestra?

Ans. Pituitary

Q-132. Bones become soft due to which disease?

Ans. Rickets

Q-133. Which substance is essential to regulate body temperature?

Ans. Water

Q-134. What is the inner concave part of the kidney called?

Ans. Hilus

Q-135. _____ are the bloood vessels which carry blood towards the heart.

Ans. Veins

Q-136. Which vein in human body alone carries pure blood?

Ans. Pulmonary vein

Q-137. The fungal derivative used in the treatment of tuberculosis is _____.

Ans. Streptomycin

Q-138. What is the outer region of the brain called?

Ans. Piamater

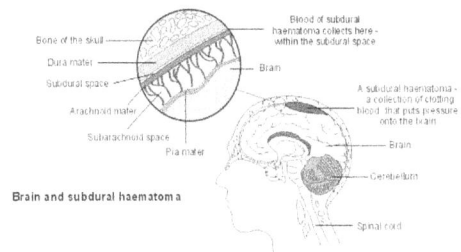

Brain and its parts

Q-139. Which body part does Poliomyelitis normally affect?

Ans. Spinal Cord

Q-140. During digestion, Protein gets converted into what?

Ans. Amino acids

Q-141. Which mineral is essential for the production of haemoglobin?

Ans. Iron

Q-142. Which mineral is necessary for the synthesis of thyroid hormones, thyroxine and triodothyronine in human body?

Ans. Iodine

Q-143. Oral zinc is used for treating _____ in children.

Ans. Diarrhea

Q-144. Who postulated the Germ Theory?

Ans. Louis Pasteur

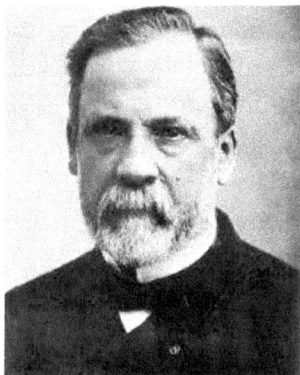

Louis Pasteur

Q-145. Serum billirubin is a causative factor of which disease?

Ans. Jaundice

Q-146. The legs of Bees covered with feather-like hairs are called _____.

Ans. Setae

Q-147. What is the female reproduction of flower consisting of ovary, stigma, and style called?

Ans. Pistil

Q-148. Which part of the plant separates vascular bundle from cortex?

Ans. Endodermis

Q-149. _____ absorbs water and nutrients into the root.

Ans. Epidermis

Q-150. The relationship between bees and sexual plants is called _____.

Ans. Symbiosis

Q-151. What tissues secrete sugar-rich nectar?

Ans. Nectaries

Q-152. Pollination by insects is described by which term?

Ans. Entomophilies

Q-153. What is a green leaf-like structure at the base of the petals protecting the developing flower called?

Ans. Sepal

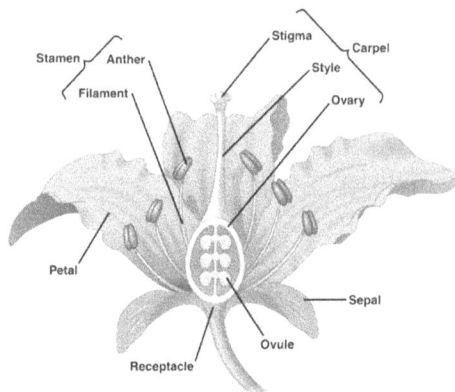

Flower reproductive system

Q-154. Meiosis occurs in anther of which plants?

Ans. Vascular plants

Q-155. What produces HCG, progesterone and estrogens?

Ans. Placenta

Q-156. What is the Stalk of ovule called?

Ans. Funicle

Q-157. How many chromosomes are there in female gamete?

Ans. 24

Q-158. Plants that are developed in dry conditions are called _____.

Ans. Xerophytes

Q-159. Photosynthesis takes place faster in which light?

Ans. White light

Q-160. Who discovered measles vaccine?

Ans. John F. Enders

Q-161. Potato is a modified form of _____.

Ans. Stem

Q-162. Which branch deals with the study of fossils?

Ans. Palaeontology

Q-163. Which kinds of plants grow best in sand?

Ans. Psammophytes

Q-164. What kinds of cells do not have a nucleus?

Ans. Prokaryote Cells

Q-165. Who proposed the theory of Biogenesis first?

Ans. Fransesco Redi

Q-166. A plant that grows in saline water is called _____.

Ans. Halophyte

Q-167. Which is a folded membrane that moves materials around in the cell?

Ans. Endoplasmic Reticulum

Q-168. Who proposed Biogenetic law?

Ans. Haeckel

Q-169. Who proposed Cosmozoic theory?

Ans. Arrhenius

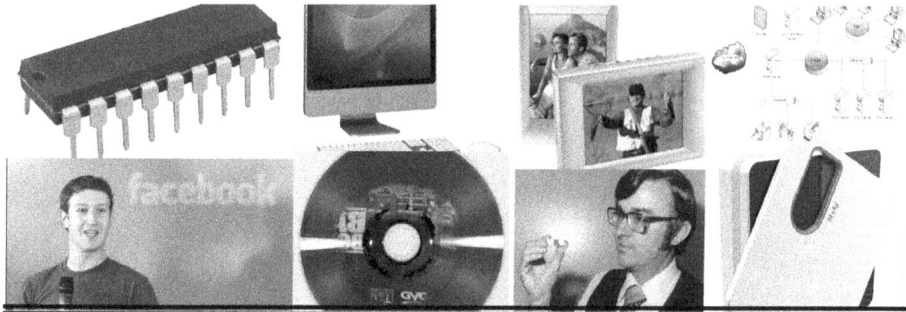

INFORMATION TECHNOLOGY

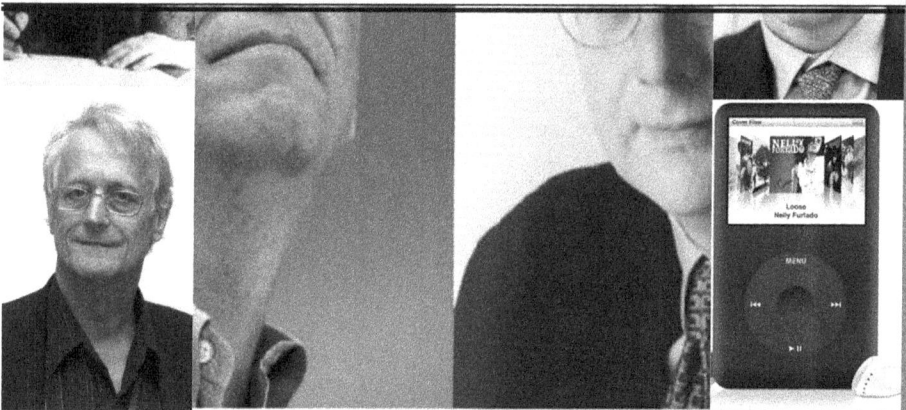

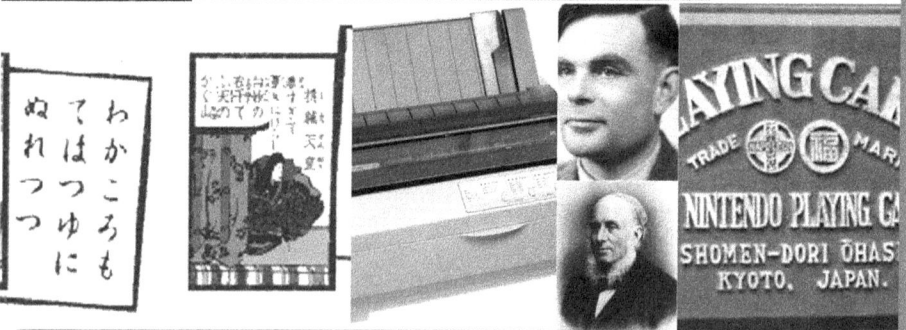

わ か こ ろ も
て は つ ゆ に
ぬ れ つ つ

NINTENDO PLAYING CA
SHOMEN-DORI ŌHAS
KYOTO, JAPAN.

Q-1. Firefox, Opera, Chrome, Safari and Explorer are types of what?

Ans. Internet Browsers

Q-2. Along with whom did Bill Gates found Microsoft?

Ans. Paul Allen

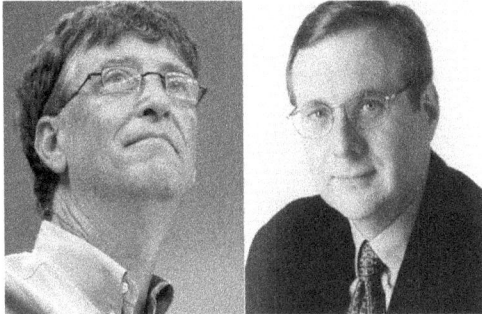

Bill Gates and Paul Allen

Q-3. What does the abbreviation WWW stand for?

Ans. World Wide Web

Q-4. One kilobyte is equal to how many bytes?

Ans. 1024 bytes

Q-5. In computers, what is Red Hat Linux?

Ans. Operating system

Q-6. Which Super Computer is made by Indian Scientists?

Ans. Param

Q-7. One Gigabyte is equal to how many bytes?

Ans. 1000,000,000 bytes approximately

Q-8. In computers, _____ are errors that can be pointed out by compilers.

Ans. Syntax errors

Q-9. What is the Control Unit's function in the CPU?

Ans. To perform Logic functions

Q-10. The command 'Ctrl + Alt + Dlt' is used for what?

Ans. To reboot the computer

Q-11. What is the full form LAN?

Ans. Local Area Network

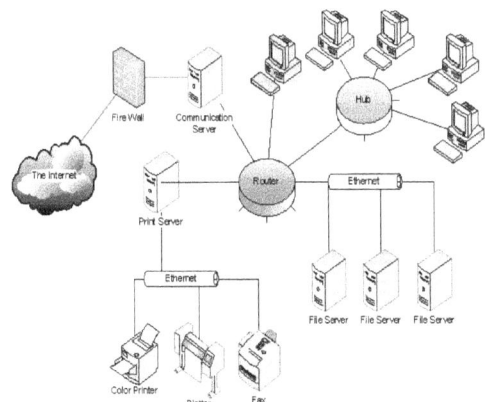

LAN structure

Q-12. Where is Silicon Valley of India located?

Ans. Bangalore

Q-13. What is ROM composed of?

Ans. Micro processors

Q-14. What is the computer code for interchange of information between terminals?

Ans. ASCII

Q-15. What is MS-DOS?

Ans. System Software

Q-16. BASIC, COBOL, FORTRAN are examples of what?

Ans. Computer language

Q-17. Who was the inventor of mechanical calculator for adding numbers?

Ans. Pascal

Q-18. Who wrote the first book on personal computers, 'Computer Liberation and Dream Machine'?

Ans. Ted Nelson

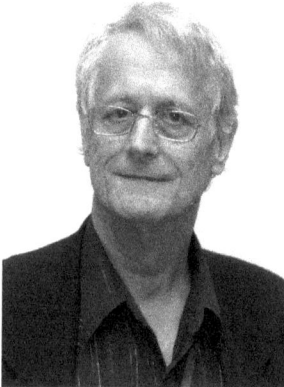

Ted Nelson

Q-19. _____ is a stored program machine.

Ans. Micro Computer

Q-20. First generation computers used _____.

Ans. Vacuum tubes

Q-21. Transistors are used with which computer system?

Ans. Second generation

Q-22. A _____ is a unit of hardware which an operator uses to monitor computer processing.

Ans. Console

Q-23. The translator program that converts source code in high level language into machine code line by line is called _____.

Ans. Translator

Q-24. Who invented Microprocessor?

Ans. Ted Hoff

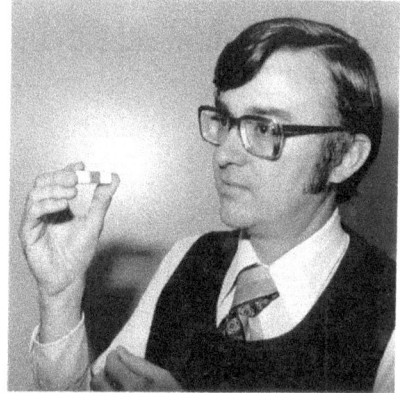

Ted Hoff

Q-25. Software that can manipulate or destroy data or programs in a computer is known as _____.

Ans. Virus

Q-26. Which computer company introduced mouse for the first time?

Ans. Apple Corporation

Q-27. Who developed the World Wide Web first?

Ans. Timothy Berners Lee

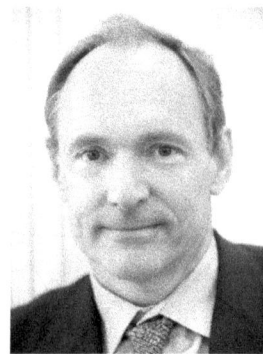

Timothy Berners Lee

Q-28. What high-level computer language was named after a French mathematician and philosopher?

Ans. PASCAL

Q-29. Which is the first large scale, general purpose digital computer?

Ans. ENIAC

Q-30. What is the full form of OS?

Ans. Operating System

Q-31. The ribbon is used in which printer?

Ans. Dot-Matrix printer

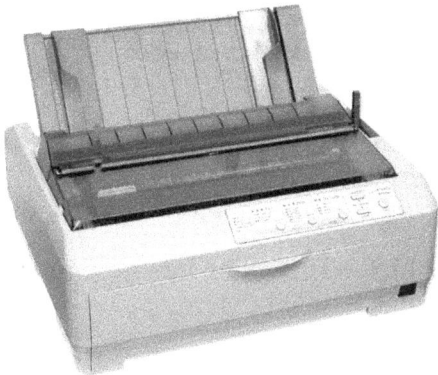

Dot Matrix Printer

Q-32. What does a DNS translate a domain name into?

Ans. Into IP

Q-33. What is IP?

Ans. Internet Protocol

Q-34. When was the first e-mail sent?

Ans. In 1971

TRIVIA

The first e-mail was sent by Ray Tomlinson in 1971.

Q-35. What type of memory is volatile?

Ans. RAM

Q-36. In computers, main memory is also known as what?

Ans. Primary memory

Q-37. What is the full Form of NIC?

Ans. Network Interface Card

TRIVIA

NIC is Network Interface Card which is used to connect a computer to a Network.

Q-38. What is the collection of communication lines and routers called?

Ans. Communication Subnet

Q-39. Which type of channels moves data relatively slowly?

Ans. Narrow band channel

Q-40. A protocol is a set of rules governing a time sequence of events that must take place between _____.

Ans. Peers

Q-41. What is the full form of HTTP?

Ans. Hyper Text Transfer Protocol

Q-42. Radio communication frequency ranges from _____.

Ans. 3 KHz to 300 GHz

Q-43. The frequency ranges from 300 KHz to 3 MHz is used for which purpose?

Ans. AM radio transmission

Q-44. What is the full form of ISP?

Ans. Internet Service Provider

Q-45. IC chips used in computers are generally made up of what?

Ans. Silicon

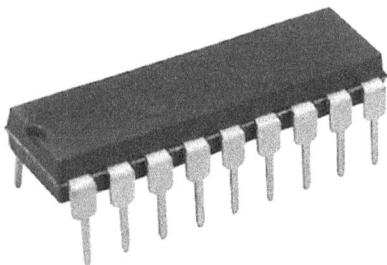

IC chips

Q-46. A concentric ring on a hard disk is referred to as a?

Ans. Track

Q-47. A computer contains many electric, electronic, and mechanical components known as _____.

Ans. Hardware

Q-48. What are the two categories of software?

Ans. System software and Application Software

Q-49. Which is the most common storage device for the personal computer?

Ans. Hard Disk Drive

Q-50. A DVD is an example of _____ .

Ans. An optical disk

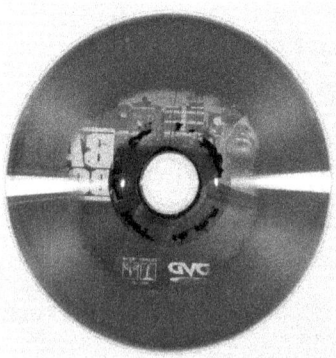

A DVD

Q-51. Users can access mail anywhere using what?

Ans. Webmail Interface

Q-52. ____is a small piece of data sent from a website and stored in a user's Hard Drive while a user is browsing a website.

Ans. Cookie

Q-53. A _____ is a set of characters that share common design features.

Ans. Typeface

Q-54. What is the process of contracting an existing business process to give another organization on other country called?

Ans. Outsource

Q-55. What is Writing, Formatting, Printing called?

Ans. Word Processing

Q-56. Method of getting Internet on Telephone line is called _____.

Ans. DSL line

Q-57. An _____ is a digital circuit that performs arithmetic and logical operations.

Ans. ALU

Q-58. Which technology allows user to upload files Online?

Ans. Webhosting technology

Q-59. The main route that data travels over the internet is called _____.

Ans. Internet backbone

Q-60. An internet protocol that allows quick file transmission to remote computers is known as _____.

Ans. FTP

Q-61. Who is the Founder of the social networking website 'Facebook'?

Ans. Mark Eliot Zuckerberg

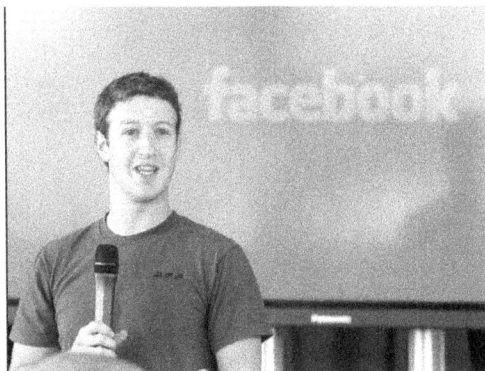

Mark Eliot Zuckerberg

Q-62. Which device protects all computers in the network from many attacks?

Ans. Firewall

Q-63. A company which maintains internet computers and telecommunications equipment in order to provide internet access to businesses organizations and individuals is called _____.

Ans. Internet Service Provider

Q-65. Worms and Trojan Horses are examples of what?

Ans. Malware

Q-66. The laser printer was invented at _____.

Ans. Xerox

Q-67. Which body standardized the original implementation of the C programming language?

Ans. ANSI

Q-68. Which is a signalling method that handles a relatively wide range of frequencies?

Ans. Broadband

Q-69. Indiscriminate sending of unsolicited bulk messages is known as what?

Ans. Spamming

Q-70. GRUB is a _____.

Ans. Boot loader

Q-71. A head crash is said to occur when the read-write head of a hard disk drive _____.

Ans. Touches the magnetic media

Q-72. Which term identifies a specific computer on the web and the main page of the entire site?

Ans. Domain name

Q-73. What is the process of finding errors in software's source code known as?

Ans. Debugging

Q-74. What does HDTV stand for?

Ans. High Definition Television

Q-75. What is the full form of GPS?

Ans. Global Positioning System

Q-76. What does GIS stand for?

Ans. Geographic Information Systems

Q-77. What is the full form of CDMA?

Ans. Code Division Multiple Access

Q-78. What does ANSI stand for?

Ans. American National Standards Institute

Q-79. An icon or animation to represent a participant used in Internet chat and games is referred to as what?

Ans. Avtar

Q-80. Which famous computer was used by British code-breakers to read encrypted German messages during World War II?

Ans. Colossus

TRIVIA

Colossus was the first wholly electronic computing device. It was used to decipher messages which had been encrypted using the German Lorenz SZ 40/42 cipher machine.

Q-81. Name the English mathematician, logician and cryptographer who is regarded as the father of modern computer science.

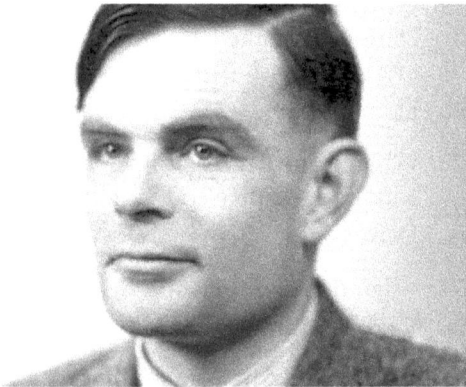

Alan Turing

Ans. Alan Turing

Q-82. This second generation computer captured a third of the world market; more than one hundred thousand units were deployed between 1960 and 1964.

Ans. IBM 1401

Q-83. Computers flourished in their third generation, thanks to Jack St. Clair Kilby and Robert Noyce's independent invention. What did they invent?

Ans. Integrated circuit (IC) or microchip

Q-84. Name the computer engineer and co-founder of Apple Computer who is often credited with developing the first mass-market home computers.

Ans. Steve "Woz" Wozniak

Q-85. Which was the first version of Microsoft Windows to support Plug and Play?

Ans. Windows 85

Q-86. What does DOS stand for?

Ans. Disk Operating System

Q-87. What does the abbreviation USB actually stand for?

Ans. Universal Serial Bus

Q-88. What does MAC stand for, when referring to computers?

Ans. Macintosh

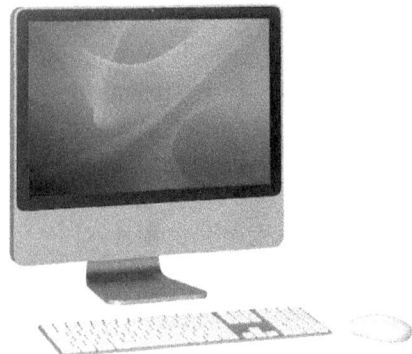

Mac

Q-89. UPS, an abbreviation referring to a piece of equipment which provides battery backup, stands for what?

Ans. Uninterruptible Power Supply

Q-90. FAT, a file system developed by Microsoft, is the shortened form of what?

Ans. File Allocation Table

Q-91. PDAs are handheld devices, helpful in handling daily schedules. What does the abbreviation PDA stand for?

Ans. Personal Digital Assistant

Q-92. Which astronomical phenomenon is also a popular programming environment?

Ans. Eclipse

Q-93. The name of which capital city also refers to an open source project for the Java platform?

Ans. Jakarta

Q-94. Which art term is also used to refer to dependencies between computer applications or processes?

Ans. Choreography

Q-95. On the Internet, who or what is a server?

Ans. The computer on which the programs of a website run.

Q-96. In the web address http://www.microsoft.com, the "com" at the end means what?

Ans. Commercial

Q-97. CQ is a type of what?

Ans. An instant messaging computer program

Q-98. Who may use the .gov domain?

Ans. US Federal Agencies

Q-99. What is the most likely suffix of a web page established by a Scottish company or individual?

Ans. .uk

Q-100. Where is the main Internet computer located?

Ans. Nowhere

Q-101. In which year did Apple's iPhone become available first?

Ans. 2007

Q-102. Nintendo was found in which year?

Ans. 1889

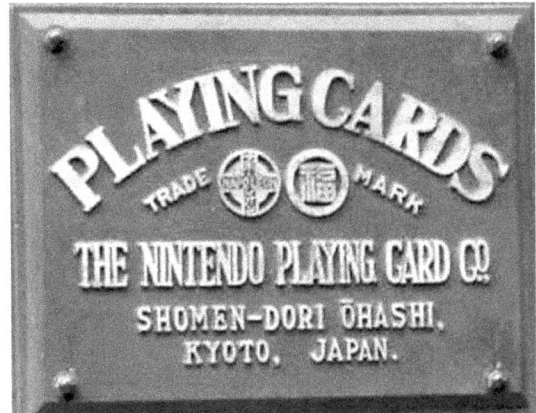

Nintendo

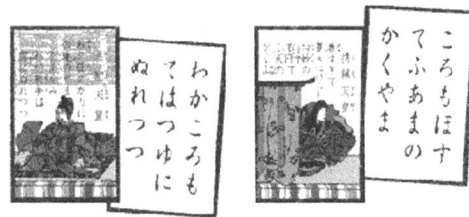

Nintendo Playing Cards

Q-103. The technologically advanced humanoid robot ASIMO is made by which car company?

Ans. Honda

Q-104. IBM is a well known computer and information technology company, what does IBM stand for?

Ans. International Business Machines

Q-105. What did the original Sony Playstation use to play games?

Ans. CDs

Q-106. Nano, Shuffle, Classic and Touch are variations of what?

Ans. Apple iPod

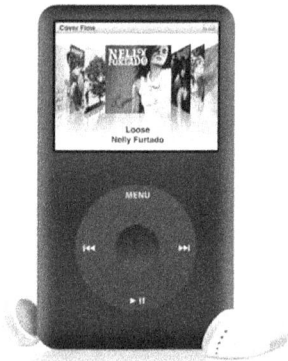

iPod

Q-107. What is the full form of ATM?

Ans. Automatic Teller Machine

Q-108. This device is the first of its kind. It balances automatically only on two wheels and is used for human transportation in pedestrian areas.

Ans. Seway HT

Q-109. Name the device that looks like an ordinary pen, but is actually a scanner.

Ans. DocuPen R-700

Q-110. This RFID-enabled digital door lock can be opened with an RFID-equipped cell phone, although it also has a slide-out keypad if you are too paranoid.

Ans. MyKey 2300

Q-111. Name the smallest VoIP phone.

Ans. The Anyuser ImPhone

Q-112. This invention works like a mobile electronic watchdog that can hear, see and even feel temperatures, thanks to its sensors.

Ans. Siemens MyAy

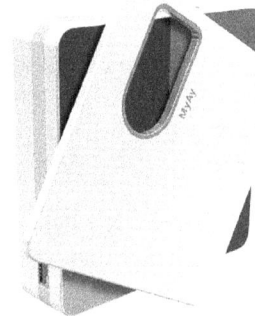

Siemens MyAy

Q-113. Name the phone that makes your QWERTY keyboard quite unnecessary. You can write down the information the old-fashioned way and this device will store it.

Ans. Siemens PenPhone

Q-114. This gadget combines a video recorder, digital camera, 128MB of data storage, web cam and a voice recorder.

Ans. Multipod 5 in 1

Q-115. Clip this gadget over the waistband of your jeans and it will record each step you make.

Ans. SportBrain Personal Fitness Manager

Q-116. Besides playing music, many such devices have voice recording capabilities and FM radio. They can recharge while transferring data to/from your computer. What is that?

Ans. MP3 Player

Q-117. This gadget is an electronic picture frame which can store 12 of your favourite images for a slide show display in any room (with an AC outlet) in your house.

Ans. Kensington Digital Photo Album

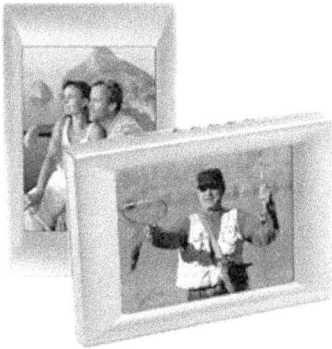

Kensington Digital Photo Album

Q-118. Who invented the blender in 1922?

Ans. Stephen Poplawski

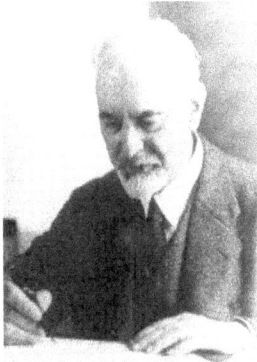

Stephen Poplawski

Q-119. Who invented the first crude metal detector?

Ans. Alexander Graham Bell

Q-120. In which year was the first remote control brought in use?

Ans. In 1956

Q-121. Who was the inventor of Fax machine?

Ans. Alexander Bain, a Scottish inventor, 1842

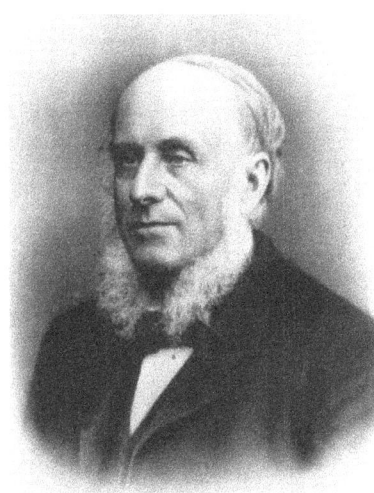

Alexander Bain

Q-122. Who patented Xerography in 1940?

Ans. Chester Carlson

Q-123. Who invented 'dishwasher'?

Ans. Josephine Cochrane in 1886

Q-124. Who was the inventor of stethoscope?

Ans. Rene Hyacinth Laennec

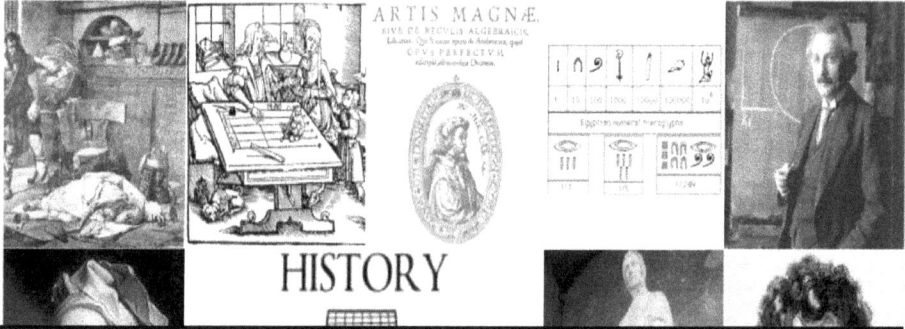

HISTORY

MATHEMATICS

of MATHEMATICS

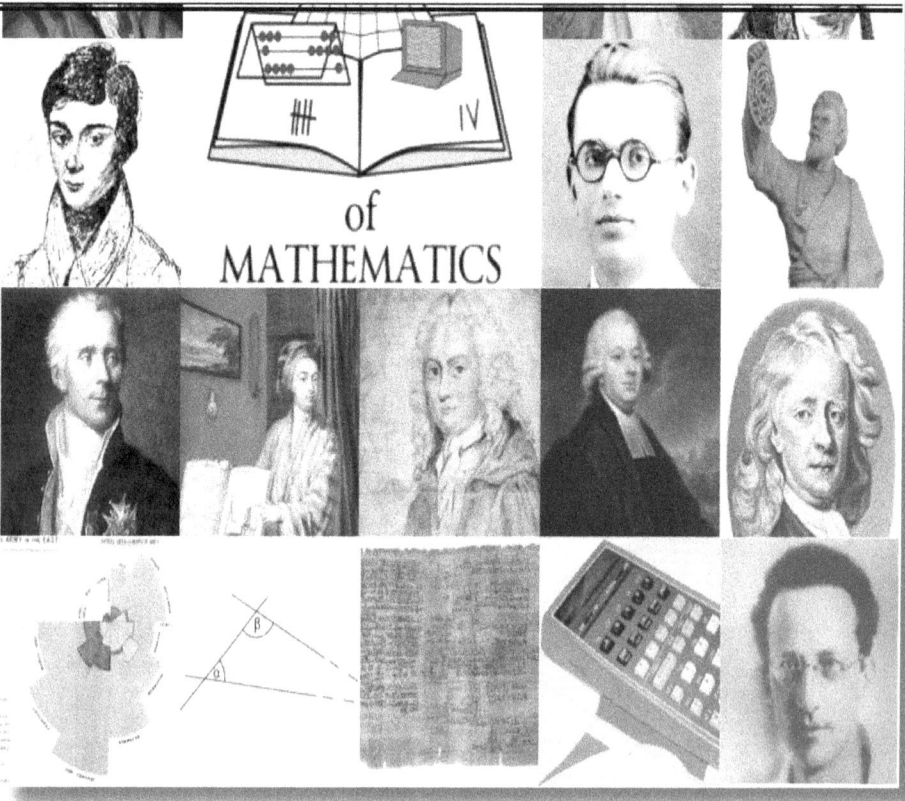

Q-1. Antonine Parent had presented his first work on analytical geometry of ____ dimensions.

    Ⓐ 2   Ⓑ 3

    Ⓒ 4   Ⓓ 5

Ans. Ⓑ

Q-2. The idea of polar co-ordinate is due to –

    Ⓐ Descartes   Ⓑ Leibnitz

    Ⓒ Gregorio Fontana Ⓓ De Moivre

Ans. Ⓒ

Q-3. Who is called the creator of vector analysis?

    Ⓐ Gauss

    Ⓑ Hermann Grassmarm

    Ⓒ Peacock

    Ⓓ Pythagoras

Ans. Ⓑ

Q-4. Which branch of mathematics had its origin from painting?

    Ⓐ Graph Theory

    Ⓑ Operational Research

    Ⓒ Projective Geometry

    Ⓓ Informative Theory

Ans. Ⓒ

Q-5. Modern analytical geometry is called Cartesian geometry on the name of –

    Ⓐ Euclid   Ⓑ Thales

    Ⓒ Descartes   Ⓓ Diophantus

Ans. Ⓒ

Q-6. The Theory of Relativity given by Einstein is based on –

    Ⓐ Euclidean Geometry

    Ⓑ Riemannian Geometry

    Ⓒ Projective Geometry

    Ⓓ Graph Theory

Ans. Ⓑ

Q-7. Who coined the new branch Functional Analysis in mathematics?

    Ⓐ Abel   Ⓑ Banach

    Ⓒ Dedekind   Ⓓ Bayes

Ans. Ⓑ

Q-8. The study of geometry and trigonometry of figures on the surface of a sphere is called –

    Ⓐ Projective geometry   Ⓑ Acturial Science

    Ⓒ Spherics   Ⓓ 3-D-Geometry

Ans. Ⓒ

Q-9. Which branch of mathematics is the system analysis associated with?

    Ⓐ Dynamics   Ⓑ Calculas

    Ⓒ Statics   Ⓓ Computer Science

Ans. Ⓓ

Q-10. Who coined the term Co-ordinate, Ordinate and Abscissa used in Analytical Geometry?

    Ⓐ Archimedes   Ⓑ Descartes

    Ⓒ Leibnitz   Ⓓ Diophantus

Ans. Ⓑ

Q-11. Who used the term commutative and distributive in the usual algebraic sense in mathematics?

    Ⓐ Hamilton   Ⓑ Newton

    Ⓒ Servois   Ⓓ Napier

Ans. Ⓒ

Q-12. Who suggested the term Linear Programming to Dantzig?

    Ⓐ I J Koopmans   Ⓑ Stigner

    Ⓒ Laderman   Ⓓ Hooper

Ans. Ⓐ

Q-13. Who coined the term Mathematical Induction in mathematics?

   Ⓐ Leibniz   Ⓑ De Morgan
   Ⓒ L' Hospital   Ⓓ Apollonous

Ans. Ⓑ

Q-14. Who coined the term Matrix in mathematics?

   Ⓐ Gauss   Ⓑ Euler
   Ⓒ Sylvester   Ⓓ Fleming

Ans. Ⓒ

Q-15. Who suggested the use of simplex method in the LPP (Linear Programming Problem)?

   Ⓐ Cayley   Ⓑ Weierestrass
   Ⓒ Dantzig   Ⓓ Sylvester

Ans. Ⓒ

Q-16. Arithmetic is derived from the word Arithmetika, what does it mean?

   Ⓐ The number theory
   Ⓑ Calculation
   Ⓒ The number science
   Ⓓ Digging earth

Ans. Ⓒ

Q-17. Percentage has the origin from the Latin word_____

   Ⓐ Percentum   Ⓑ Percentium
   Ⓒ Percenti   Ⓓ Permutation

Ans. Ⓐ

Q-18. How many digits are there in the Hindu-Arabic system?

   Ⓐ 10   Ⓑ 20
   Ⓒ 30   Ⓓ 40

Ans. Ⓐ

Q-19. What is the smallest Natural number?

   Ⓐ 1   Ⓑ 0
   Ⓒ −1   Ⓓ 10100

Ans. Ⓐ

Q-20. What is the smallest Whole number?

   Ⓐ 1   Ⓑ 0
   Ⓒ −1   Ⓓ 10^{100}

Ans. Ⓑ

Q-21. Among the following, which natural number has no predecessor?

   Ⓐ 100   Ⓑ 1
   Ⓒ 1729   Ⓓ googal

Ans. Ⓑ

Q-22. Which among the following is the largest known number in the world?

   Ⓐ ∞   Ⓑ googal
   Ⓒ googalplex   Ⓓ crore

Ans. Ⓒ

Q-23. Counting numbers are kept under:

   Ⓐ Natural Number
   Ⓑ Whole Number
   Ⓒ Rational Number
   Ⓓ Real Number

Ans. Ⓐ

Q-24. An integer that is divisible by 2 is called:

   Ⓐ Even Number
   Ⓑ Natural Number
   Ⓒ Odd Number
   Ⓓ Whole Number

Ans. Ⓐ

Q-25. A set of numbers which include 0 and the counting number is called:

   Ⓐ Even Number
   Ⓑ Natural Number
   Ⓒ Odd Number
   Ⓓ Whole Number

Ans. Ⓓ

Q-26. The whole number is denoted by –

- Ⓐ N
- Ⓑ R
- Ⓒ W
- Ⓓ Q

Ans. Ⓒ

Q-27. All counting numbers, together with their negatives and zero constitute the set of:

- Ⓐ Whole Number
- Ⓑ Real Number
- Ⓒ Integers
- Ⓓ Odd Number

Ans. Ⓒ

Q-28. Where was the idea of zero invented?

- Ⓐ America
- Ⓑ Europe
- Ⓒ India
- Ⓓ Italy

Ans. Ⓒ

Q-29. The method to find the primes between two numbers was given by:

- Ⓐ Einstein
- Ⓑ Euler
- Ⓒ Eratosthenes
- Ⓓ Wilson

Ans. Ⓒ

Q-30. If the sum of cubes of each digits of a number is equal to the number itself, the number is called:

- Ⓐ Kaprekar Number
- Ⓑ Lucas Number
- Ⓒ Armstrong Number
- Ⓓ Square Number

Ans. Ⓒ

Q-31. A number is called...... number if it is equal to the sum of all of its factors, except itself.

- Ⓐ Kaprekar Number
- Ⓑ Defective Number
- Ⓒ Perfect Number
- Ⓓ Cardinal Number

Ans. Ⓒ

Q-32. A number 'n' is called abundant if the sum of all of its divisors is more than:

- Ⓐ 2n
- Ⓑ 2n
- Ⓒ n^2
- Ⓓ 22n

Ans. Ⓐ

Q-33. Which among the following is the first abundant number?

- Ⓐ 12
- Ⓑ 220
- Ⓒ 1729
- Ⓓ 945

Ans. Ⓐ

Q-34. The smallest odd abundant number is:

- Ⓐ 1945
- Ⓑ 5000
- Ⓒ 1937
- Ⓓ 945

Ans. Ⓓ

Q-35. p and e are:

- Ⓐ Happy Numbers
- Ⓑ Sad Numbers
- Ⓒ Transcendental Numbers
- Ⓓ Algebraic Numbers

Ans. Ⓒ

Q-36. Number of the type $F^n = 2^{2^n} + 1$ is called:

- Ⓐ Fermat Number
- Ⓑ Kaprekar Number
- Ⓒ Fibonacci Number
- Ⓓ Happy Number

Ans. Ⓐ

Q-37. Which among the following is the largest even prime number?

- Ⓐ 2
- Ⓑ 3
- Ⓒ 8
- Ⓓ 0

Ans. Ⓐ

Q-38. What is the smallest odd prime number?

- Ⓐ 2
- Ⓑ 3
- Ⓒ 9
- Ⓓ 11

Ans. Ⓑ

Q-39. What does LCD stand for –

   Ⓐ Low Cost Depot

   Ⓑ Lower Coded Decimal

   Ⓒ Least Common Denominator

   Ⓓ Liberal Criminal Department

Ans. Ⓒ

Q-40. Which among the following is known as Beast number or Devil's number?

   Ⓐ 945   Ⓑ 6174

   Ⓒ 666   Ⓓ 2157

Ans. Ⓓ

Q-41. Which number is shown by the prefix "Uni"

   Ⓐ 0   Ⓑ 1

   Ⓒ 10   Ⓓ 2

Ans. Ⓑ

Q-42. 1 mile = ... km.

   Ⓐ 10   Ⓑ 1.254

   Ⓒ 1.6093   Ⓓ 330

Ans. Ⓐ

Q-43. 1 inch =........... centimetre.

   Ⓐ 2.54   Ⓑ 0.99

   Ⓒ 1.6093   Ⓓ 643

Ans. Ⓓ

Q-44. How many times in a day are the hands of a clock straight?

   Ⓐ 12   Ⓑ 22

   Ⓒ 24   Ⓓ 44

Ans. Ⓒ

Q-45. How many times are the hands of a clock at 90^0 in a day?

   Ⓐ 24   Ⓑ 36

   Ⓒ 44   Ⓓ 12

Ans. Ⓒ

Q-46. How many times do the hands of a clock coincide in a day?

   Ⓐ 24   Ⓑ 22

   Ⓒ 20   Ⓓ 21

Ans. Ⓑ

Q-47. How many times do the hands of a clock point towards each other in a day?

   Ⓐ 24   Ⓑ 20

   Ⓒ 22   Ⓓ 21

Ans. Ⓒ

Q-48. Which among the following is the greatest 3-digit greatest square?

   Ⓐ 100   Ⓑ 961

   Ⓒ 141   Ⓓ 396

Ans. Ⓑ

Q-49. Any two consecutive primes which differ by 2 are known as:

   Ⓐ Prime Doublet

   Ⓑ Twin Primes

   Ⓒ Mersenne Primes

   Ⓓ Co-prime

Ans. Ⓑ

Q-50. How many numbers are there between 1 and 100 that are both square and cubic?

   Ⓐ 8   Ⓑ 5

   Ⓒ 4   Ⓓ 2

Ans. Ⓓ

Q-51. How many symbols do we use in a binary code number?

   Ⓐ 2   Ⓑ 3

   Ⓒ 8   Ⓓ 16

Ans. Ⓐ

Q-52. Which among the following is the smallest perfect number?

- Ⓐ 28
- Ⓑ 424
- Ⓒ 6
- Ⓓ 3

Ans. Ⓒ

Q-53. The largest cube in the Fibonacci sequence is:

- Ⓐ 27
- Ⓑ 64
- Ⓒ 1331
- Ⓓ 9

Ans. Ⓓ

Q-54. What is the least number that can be expressed as the sum of cubes of the first two numbers?

- Ⓐ 8
- Ⓑ 9
- Ⓒ 1729
- Ⓓ 6174

Ans. Ⓑ

Q-55. What is the sum of the square of the first two odd numbers?

- Ⓐ 10
- Ⓑ 20
- Ⓒ 30
- Ⓓ 40

Ans. Ⓐ

Q-56. In which numeral system, there is no symbol for zero –

- Ⓐ Hindi-Arabic system
- Ⓑ Greeks
- Ⓒ Roman Numeral system
- Ⓓ International system

Ans. Ⓒ

Q-57. What is the sum of the first 100 natural numbers?

- Ⓐ 5000
- Ⓑ 5050
- Ⓒ 10000
- Ⓓ 100

Ans. Ⓑ

Q-58. What is the sum of the first 20 even numbers?

- Ⓐ 400
- Ⓑ 420
- Ⓒ 395
- Ⓓ 470

Ans. Ⓑ

Q-59. Which of the following are Happy numbers?

- Ⓐ 19
- Ⓑ 28
- Ⓒ 35
- Ⓓ 65

Ans. Ⓐ

Q-60. A number that is divisible by the sum of its digits is called:

- Ⓐ Ramanujan Number
- Ⓑ Harshad Number
- Ⓒ Archimedes Number
- Ⓓ Platonic Number

Ans. Ⓑ

Q-61. The fear of 13 is called:

- Ⓐ Triskaidekaphobia
- Ⓑ Claustrophobia
- Ⓒ Xenobhobia
- Ⓓ Hydrophobia

Ans. Ⓐ

Q-62. Which civilisation used the sexagesmial system in mathematics?

- Ⓐ Egyptian
- Ⓑ Babylonian
- Ⓒ Indus
- Ⓓ Italian

Ans. Ⓐ

Q-63. Who discovered the Irrational Number?

- Ⓐ Pythogoras
- Ⓑ Plato
- Ⓒ Pappus
- Ⓓ Aristotle

Ans. Ⓐ

Q-64. In Vigesimal system, the base is taken as:

- **A** 2
- **B** 3
- **C** 20
- **D** 4

Ans. **C**

Q-65. Which book of Plato deals with the Mystic number?

- **A** Theaetetus
- **B** Platonicus
- **C** Republic
- **D** Principia

Ans. **C**

Q-66. Which number is equal to the cube of the sum of its digits?

- **A** 1729
- **B** 15625
- **C** 4913
- **D** 1728

Ans. **C**

Q-67. Which two digit numbers is equal to the area and perimeter of a square?

- **A** 16
- **B** 25
- **C** 36
- **D** 64

Ans. **A**

Q-68. A number system which has its base 8 is called?

- **A** Octal Number
- **B** Hexagonal Number
- **C** Quibinary
- **D** Octagon Number

Ans. **A**

Q-69. The greatest number in Rigveda is –

- **A** 10^{12}
- **B** 10^6
- **C** 60099
- **D** 74532

Ans. **C**

Q-70. The highest number mentioned in Yajurveda is

- **A** 10^{12}
- **B** 10^{100}
- **C** 10^{18}
- **D** 10^7

Ans. **A**

Q-71. The sum of the angles of a hexagon is:

- **A** 420°
- **B** 360°
- **C** 720°
- **D** 270°

Ans. **C**

Q-72. The sum of the external angle of an octagon is:

- **A** 360°
- **B** 180°
- **C** 720°
- **D** 270°

Ans. **A**

Q-72. Who is called the Father of Geometry?

- **A** Pythagros
- **B** Euclid
- **C** Pappus
- **D** Euler

Ans. **B**

Q-73. If the sum of two angles is 90 , they are.... angles.

- **A** Complementary
- **B** Supplementary
- **C** Adjacent
- **D** Alternate

Ans. **A**

Q-74. Two angles, whose sum is 180 are called………. angles.

- **A** Complementary
- **B** Supplementary
- **C** Adjacent
- **D** Alternate

Ans. **B**

Q-75. The .... angles are two angles whose sum is 360 degrees.

- **A** Conjugate angle
- **B** Reflex angle
- **C** Acute angle
- **D** Obtuse angle

Ans. **A**

Q-76. The space between any two radii is called……….

- **A** Segment
- **B** Sector
- **C** Chord
- **D** Secant

Ans. **B**

Q-77. How many circles can be drawn through 3 non-collinear points.

Ⓐ 1   Ⓑ 2
Ⓒ 3   Ⓓ Many

Ans. Ⓐ

Q-78. Angle measure of a semi-circle is..........

Ⓐ 45°   Ⓑ 90°
Ⓒ 180°   Ⓓ 360°

Ans. Ⓑ

Q-79. The sum of either pair of opposite angles of a cyclic quadrilateral is:

Ⓐ 90°   Ⓑ 180°
Ⓒ 270°   Ⓓ 360°

Ans. Ⓑ

Q-80. The longest chord of a circle is a .... of the circle.

Ⓐ Tangent   Ⓑ Secant
Ⓒ Arc   Ⓓ Diameter

Ans. Ⓓ

Q-81. The sum of all the exterior angle of a polygon is –

Ⓐ 180°   Ⓑ 360°
Ⓒ 540°   Ⓓ 720°

Ans. Ⓑ

Q-82. The line joining the midpoint of a side to its opposite vertex is called the ......

Ⓐ centroid   Ⓑ mean
Ⓒ median   Ⓓ orthocentre

Ans. Ⓒ

Q-83. Points lying on the same line are called:

Ⓐ intersecting points
Ⓑ collinear points
Ⓒ coincidents
Ⓓ contact points

Ans. Ⓑ

Q-84. Points which lie on a common circle are:

Ⓐ Concyclic points
Ⓑ Collinear points
Ⓒ Concurrent points
Ⓓ Tangents of circle

Ans. Ⓐ

Q-85. What is the measure of each angle of Regular Octagon?

Ⓐ 120°   Ⓑ 150°
Ⓒ 140°   Ⓓ 135°

Ans. Ⓓ

Q-86. Which of the following is not the axiom of congruency of two triangles?

Ⓐ SSS   Ⓑ RHS
Ⓒ SA   Ⓓ LHS

Ans. Ⓓ

Q-87. What is the measure of each angle of an Equilateral Triangle?

Ⓐ 40°   Ⓑ 75°
Ⓒ 60°   Ⓓ 35°

Ans. Ⓒ

Q-88. A figure having 14 faces with triangle and square is known as.............

Ⓐ dodecagon
Ⓑ cube
Ⓒ cuboctahedron
Ⓓ Icosidodecahedron

Ans. Ⓒ

Q-89. A figure having 32 faces with triangles and pentagons is called.............

Ⓐ dodecagon
Ⓑ cube
Ⓒ cuboctahedron
Ⓓ Icosidodecahedron

Ans. Ⓒ

Q-90. Which of the following is not true for a square?

   Ⓐ It is a rectangle with equal sides.
   Ⓑ The diagonals bisect at 90°.
   Ⓒ The diagonals are not equal.
   Ⓓ Its perimeter is 4 times the side.

Ans. Ⓒ

Q-91. Two angles having a common side and common vertex and lying on opposite sides of their common side are called…………..

   Ⓐ Adjacent angles   Ⓑ Acute angles
   Ⓒ Alternate angles   Ⓓ Linear pairs

Ans. Ⓒ

Q-92. Which among the following theorem is also known as BPT (Basic Proportionality Theorem)?

   Ⓐ Pythagoras Theorem
   Ⓑ Wilson Theorem
   Ⓒ Congruence Theorem
   Ⓓ Thales Theorem

Ans. Ⓓ

Q-93. Which of the following is the Cartesian Equation of asteroid curve?

   Ⓐ $x^{2/3} + y^{2/3} = a^{2/3}$
   Ⓑ $r = a^2\theta$
   Ⓒ $x^2 + y^2 = r^2$
   Ⓓ $\dfrac{x^2}{a^2} + \dfrac{y^2}{b^2} = 1$

Ans. Ⓐ

Q-94. Which of the following represents a circle?

   Ⓐ $\dfrac{x^2}{a^2} + \dfrac{y^2}{b^2} = 1$ Ⓑ $\dfrac{x^2}{a^2} - \dfrac{y^2}{b^2} = 1$
   Ⓒ $(x-b)^2 + (y-k)^2 = r^2$
   Ⓓ $x^{2/3} + y^{2/3} = 1$

Ans. Ⓒ

Q-95. Which of the following represents the equation of a Catenary?

   Ⓐ $y = x^2 + r^2$
   Ⓑ $r = 2a(1 + \cos\theta)$
   Ⓒ $y = a \cos h \dfrac{x}{a}$
   Ⓓ $x = a \cos^2 t$

Ans. Ⓒ

Q-96. The Parametric Equation of circle is:

   Ⓐ $x = a \cos^3 t, y = a \sin^3 t$
   Ⓑ $x = t - 1, y = t^2 + 1$
   Ⓒ $x = \sin\theta, y = a \cos\theta$
   Ⓓ $x = o \ s^3\theta$

Ans. Ⓒ

Q-97. If p is prime then 1+(p-1)! is divisible by p, whose statement is this?

   Ⓐ Waring   Ⓑ Goldbich
   Ⓒ Fermat   Ⓓ Wilson

Ans. Ⓓ

Q-98. The Fundamental Theorem of Algebra that "Every m degree polynomial has m roots" was proved by-

    Ⓐ Euler   Ⓑ Gauss

    Ⓒ Galois   Ⓓ Gunter

Ans. Ⓑ

Q-99. To whom is the first theorem relating to circles attributed?

    Ⓐ Thales   Ⓑ Pythagoras

    Ⓒ Apollonius   Ⓓ Agnesi

Ans. Ⓐ

Q-100. Which law is followed by the bee in building the wax cells of honey comb?

    Ⓐ Maxima and Minima

    Ⓑ Gravitational law

    Ⓒ Algebraic law

    Ⓓ Law of large numbers

Ans. Ⓐ

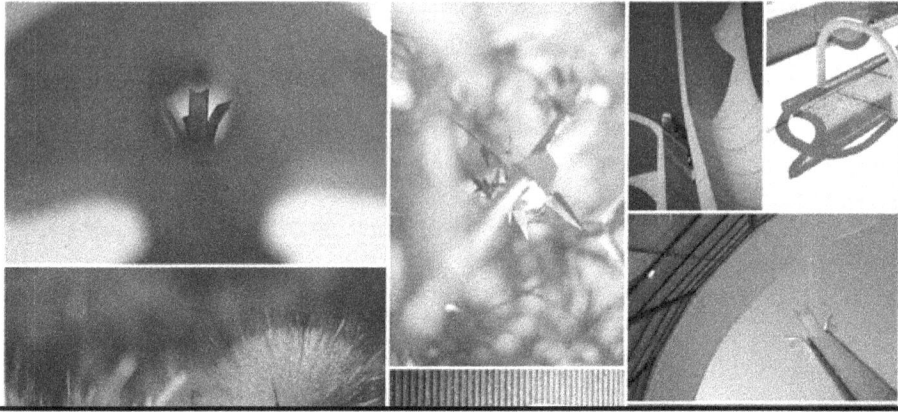

ENVIRONMENT

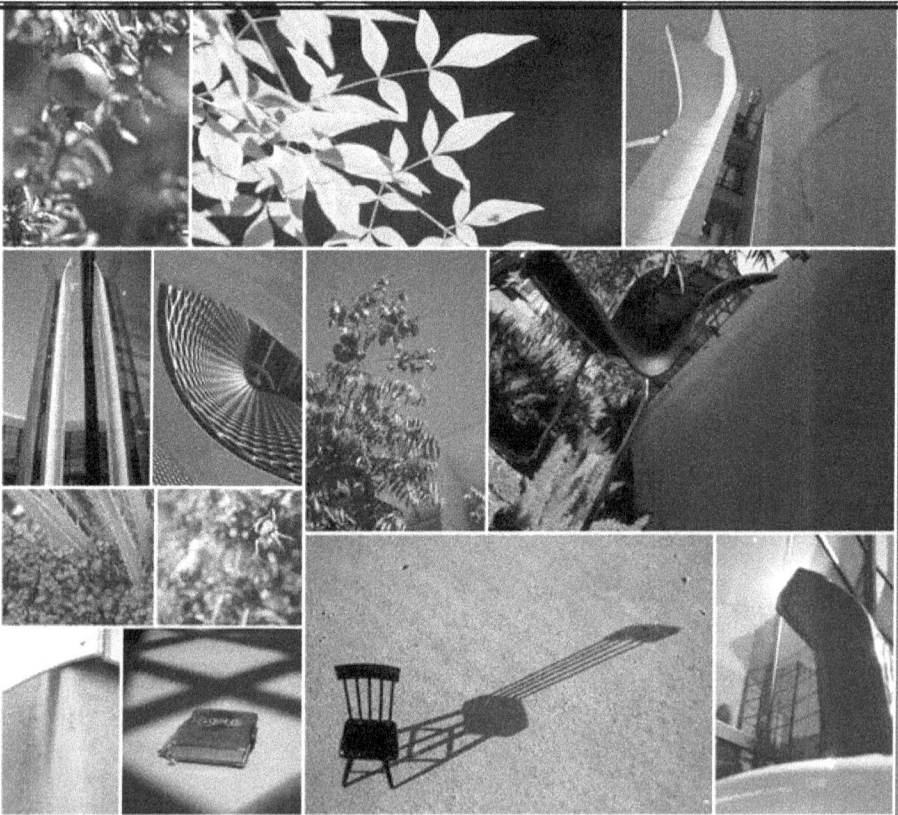

Q-1. Which of the following chemicals is present in acid rain?
- **a** Sulphuric acid
- **b** Paraffin wax
- **c** Carbon dioxide
- **d** Aluminium

Ans. **a**

Q-2. Which of the following substances is non-biodegradable?
- **a** Plastic
- **b** Manure
- **c** Paper
- **d** Wood

Ans. **a**

Q-3. The Kaziranga Sanctuary is located in:
- **a** Lucknow
- **b** Bhopal
- **c** Manipur
- **d** Assam

Ans. **d**

Q-4. El Nino is the name of:
- **a** An extinct animal
- **b** A motor vehicle
- **c** A weather current
- **d** A hurricane

Ans. **c**

Q-5. Which of the following is not an Indian biosphere reserve?
- **a** Sunderbans
- **b** Nilgiri
- **c** Gulf of Mannar
- **d** Gulf of Kachh

Ans. **d**

Q-6. The Sandalwood tree can be found in a/an:
- **a** Deciduous forest
- **b** Deltaic forest
- **c** Evergreen forest
- **d** Thorny forest

Ans. **a**

Q-7. The Alluvial soil is deposited by:
- **a** Rivers and streams
- **b** Wind
- **c** Rain
- **d** Living organisms

Ans. **a**

Q-8. Black soil lacks:
- **a** Iron
- **b** Phosphorus
- **c** Magnesia
- **d** Alumina

Ans. **b**

Q-9. Arid soil is:
- **a** Red or brown in colour
- **b** Yellow in colour
- **c** Deep grey in colour
- **d** Black in colour

Ans. **a**

Q-10. Which of the following gases was mainly responsible for the Bhopal Gas Tragedy?
- **a** Methyl isocyanate
- **b** Methane
- **c** Sulphur dioxide
- **d** Carbon dioxide

Ans. **a**

Q-11. The Bhopal Gas Tragedy took place on:
- **a** December 3, 1984
- **b** October 5, 1996
- **c** December 3, 1996
- **d** October 5, 1984

Ans. **a**

Q-12. In which gas plant did the Bhopal Gas Tragedy take place?
- **a** Hindustan Mint and Agro Products
- **b** Union Carbide (India) Ltd
- **c** Pacific Agricorp Pvt Ltd
- **d** Dow Chemical Co

Ans. **b**

Q-13. The annual rate of continent drifting is:

    ⓐ 15 to 16 cm   ⓒ 20 to 75 mm
    ⓑ 17 to 18 inches   ⓓ 1 to 2 km

Ans. ⓒ

Q-14. The last Ice Age took place:

    ⓐ 200 million years ago
    ⓑ 1500 years ago
    ⓒ 18,000 years ago
    ⓓ 16 million years ago

Ans. ⓒ

Q-15. Earthquakes take place due to:

    ⓐ Movement in tectonic plates
    ⓑ Global warming
    ⓒ Habitat destruction
    ⓓ Change in weather

Ans. ⓐ

Q-16. The Earth's outer crust is divided into:

    ⓐ Seven large tectonic plates
    ⓑ 16 large tectonic plates
    ⓒ Two tectonic plates
    ⓓ Innumerable plates

Ans. ⓐ

Q-17. During a shift/collision in the tectonic plates, the energy is released in the form of:

    ⓐ Radiation
    ⓑ Sound waves
    ⓒ Seismic waves
    ⓓ Ultraviolet radiation

Ans. ⓒ

Q-18. The intensity of an earthquake is measured on a:

    ⓐ Richter scale   ⓒ Ammeter
    ⓑ Speedometer   ⓓ Volt meter

Ans. ⓐ

Q-19. Who said these words: "Poverty is the worst form of pollution..."

    ⓐ Rajiv Gandhi
    ⓑ Jawaharlal Nehru
    ⓒ Indira Gandhi
    ⓓ Mahatma Gandhi

Ans. ⓒ

Q-20. The Big Bang is a theory about:

    ⓐ A car accident
    ⓑ A nuclear radiation leak
    ⓒ The beginning of the universe
    ⓓ An atomic bomb explosion

Ans. ⓒ

Q-21. A light year is a unit used to measure:

    ⓐ Radiation   ⓑ Brightness
    ⓒ Time   ⓓ Distance

Ans. ⓓ

Q-22. The closest star to the earth is:

    ⓐ Mercury   ⓑ Moon
    ⓒ Sun   ⓓ Pluto

Ans. ⓒ

Q-23. Ocean basins are made of:

    ⓐ Basaltic rock   ⓑ Granite rock
    ⓒ Silicates   ⓓ Phosphates

Ans. ⓐ

Q-24. The landmass of the earth (continents) is made up of:

    ⓐ Basaltic rock   ⓑ Granite rock
    ⓒ Silicates   ⓓ Phosphates

Ans. ⓑ

Q-25. Granite rocks are made of:

    ⓐ Calcium sulphate

    ⓑ Sodium chloride

    ⓒ Aluminium silicate

    ⓓ Phosphates

Ans. ⓒ

Q-26. Basaltic rocks are made of:

    ⓐ Calcium sulphate

    ⓑ Magnesium silicate

    ⓒ Aluminium phosphate

    ⓓ Aluminium silicate

Ans. ⓑ

Q-27. The first life form to appear on the earth was:

    ⓐ Man

    ⓒ Cactus plant

    ⓑ Dinosaur

    ⓓ Blue-green algae

Ans. ⓓ

Q-28. How many layers does soil have?

    ⓐ One   ⓑ Two

    ⓒ Three   ⓓ Four

Ans. ⓒ

Q-29. Hydrosphere does not consist of:

    ⓐ Oceans   ⓑ Rainwater

    ⓒ Glaciers   ⓓ Lakes

Ans. ⓑ

Q-30. The carbon dioxide level in the atmosphere is directly related to:

    ⓐ The earth's temperature

    ⓑ The type of vegetation

    ⓒ Water scarcity

    ⓓ Soil erosion

Ans. ⓐ

Q-31. Lightning during rains is a form of:

    ⓐ Thunder

    ⓑ Electric discharge

    ⓒ Sound release

    ⓓ Bright clouds

Ans. ⓑ

Q-32. The speed of light is:

    ⓐ Faster than the speed of sound

    ⓑ Slower than the speed of sound

    ⓒ One-eighth the speed of sound

    ⓓ Equal to the speed of sound

Ans. ⓐ

Q-33. Blue-agree algae appeared:

    ⓐ On the landmass

    ⓑ In the atmosphere

    ⓒ Around trees

    ⓓ On the surface of the ocean

Ans. ⓓ

Q-34. The last living organism to appear on earth was:

    ⓐ Blue whale   ⓑ Dolphin

    ⓒ Humans   ⓓ Birds

Ans. ⓒ

Q-35. The geological cycle means:

    ⓐ Recycling of the earth's crust

    ⓑ Change in the geographical features of a region

    ⓒ The constant movement of carbon in the atmosphere

    ⓓ The constant movement of living beings from one place to another

Ans. ⓐ

Q-36. Plants give off excess water through the process of:

- ⓐ Respiration
- ⓑ Transpiration
- ⓒ Evaporation
- ⓓ Condensation

Ans. ⓑ

Q-37. One major cause of eutrophication is:

- ⓐ Phosphate pollution of water
- ⓒ Excess carbon in water
- ⓑ Chlorine pollution of water
- ⓓ Sulphate pollution in water

Ans. ⓐ

Q-38. Rocks formed after cooling of molten lava are called:

- ⓐ Granite rocks
- ⓑ Igneous rocks
- ⓒ Sedimentary rocks
- ⓓ Glaciers

Ans. ⓑ

Q-39. The Tundra biome is in the:

- ⓐ Tropical region
- ⓑ Equatorial region
- ⓒ Polar region
- ⓓ Desert region

Ans. ⓒ

Q-40. Pine trees are found in:

- ⓐ Deciduous forests
- ⓑ Coniferous forests
- ⓒ Deserts
- ⓓ Polar region

Ans. ⓑ

Q-41. Tropical rainforests are found near the:

- ⓐ Equator
- ⓑ North Pole
- ⓒ South Pole
- ⓓ Desert region

Ans. ⓐ

Q-42. Marine water has high amount of:

- ⓐ Phosphates
- ⓑ Carbon
- ⓒ Salt
- ⓓ Nitrates

Ans. ⓒ

Q-43. Mangroves are:

- ⓐ A variety of mangoes
- ⓑ Forests found between land and sea
- ⓒ A variety of fish food
- ⓓ None of these

Ans. ⓑ

Q-44. The habitat of the Royal Bengal Tiger is:

- ⓐ The Sahara Desert
- ⓑ The Kaziranga National Park
- ⓒ The Sunderbans
- ⓓ None of these

Ans. ⓒ

Q-45. In India, forests are mainly cut down for:

- ⓐ Firewood (fuel)
- ⓑ Paper making
- ⓒ Furniture industry
- ⓓ Timber

Ans. ⓐ

Q-46. Which of the following is not a freshwater ecosystem?

- ⓐ Ponds
- ⓑ Lakes
- ⓒ Springs
- ⓓ Seas

Ans. ⓓ

Q-47. Green plants make their own food, hence they are:

- ⓐ Autotrophic
- ⓑ Heterotrophic
- ⓒ Consumers
- ⓓ Secondary consumers

Ans. ⓐ

Q-48. Which of the following elements is common in all the ecosystems on the earth?

    ⓐ The sun   ⓑ The moon

    ⓒ Soil   ⓓ Man

Ans. ⓐ

Q-49. Transpiration is a phenomenon that takes place in:

    ⓐ Birds

    ⓑ Plants

    ⓒ Aquatic animals

    ⓓ Humans

Ans. ⓑ

Q-50. Human beings first appeared on earth:

    ⓐ 3.5 billion years ago

    ⓑ 5 million years ago

    ⓒ 1 billion years ago

    ⓓ In 3000 B C

Ans. ⓑ

Q-51. When human-induced activities produce noise that interfere with marine mammals' communication, navigation, etc., the phenomenon is called:

    ⓐ Noise pollution

    ⓑ Noise trauma

    ⓒ Marine pollution

    ⓓ Masking

Ans. ⓓ

Q-52. Which of the following is not an example of noise pollution?

    ⓐ Masking   ⓑ Noise trauma

    ⓒ Blast trauma   ⓓ Deforestation

Ans. ⓓ

Q-53. For which of the following does the Doppler Effect not apply to?

    ⓐ Sound waves

    ⓑ Water ripples

    ⓒ Electromagnetic waves

    ⓓ Carbon dating

Ans. ⓓ

Q-54. Which of the following produces the loudest noise?

    ⓐ A dog barking

    ⓑ A vacuum cleaner

    ⓒ A jet plane taking off

    ⓓ A chain saw

Ans. ⓒ

Q-55. Which of the following is the time period required for a country's population to grow double?

    ⓐ Fertility rate

    ⓑ Mortality rate

    ⓒ Light year

    ⓓ Doubling time

Ans. ⓓ

Q-56. Overpopulation directly affects the:

    ⓐ Carrying capacity of a region

    ⓑ Pollution

    ⓒ Ozone layer

    ⓓ Noise pollution

Ans. ⓐ

Q-57. Pedology is the study of:

    ⓐ Feet   ⓑ Children diet

    ⓒ Soil   ⓓ Forest cover

Ans. ⓒ

Q-58. Leaching helps in:
- ⓐ Soil formation
- ⓑ Continent drifting
- ⓒ Transpiration
- ⓓ Photosynthesis

Ans. ⓐ

Q-59. Offensive odours produced by small or big-scale industries have given rise to:
- ⓐ Odour pollution
- ⓑ Bad breath
- ⓒ Body odour
- ⓓ None of these

Ans. ⓐ

Q-60. Which of the following gases is not present in biogas?
- ⓐ Methane
- ⓑ Carbon dioxide
- ⓒ Sulphur dioxide
- ⓓ Hydrogen sulphide

Ans. ⓒ

Q-61. Which of the following cannot be used to produce biogas?
- ⓐ Manure
- ⓑ Kitchen waste
- ⓒ Plastic bottles
- ⓓ Decayed plants

Ans. ⓒ

Q-62. A mixture of gases produced within a landfill due to the action of certain microorganisms is called:
- ⓐ Greenhouse gas
- ⓑ Methane
- ⓒ Landfill gas
- ⓓ None of these

Ans. ⓒ

Q-63. Which of the following is not a fossil fuel?
- ⓐ Coal
- ⓑ Petroleum
- ⓒ Biogas
- ⓓ Natural gas

Ans. ⓒ

Q-64. Sandstone turns into _____ through tectonic compression and heating.
- ⓐ Quartzite rock
- ⓑ Quartz
- ⓒ Charcoal
- ⓓ Opal

Ans. ⓐ

Q-65. Which of the following is not a mining-related disease?
- ⓐ AIDS
- ⓑ Silicosis
- ⓒ Pneumoconiosis
- ⓓ Asbestosis

Ans. ⓐ

Q-66. Which of the following is also known as miner's lung disease?
- ⓐ Silicosis
- ⓑ Pneumoconiosis
- ⓒ Asbestosis
- ⓓ None of these

Ans. ⓑ

Q-67. Old, abandoned mines which have no oxygen are called:
- ⓐ Canyons
- ⓑ Caves
- ⓒ Blackdamp
- ⓓ Sinkholes

Ans. ⓒ

Q-68. Which disease is also known as Potter's rot?
- ⓐ Silicosis
- ⓒ Pneumoconiosis
- ⓑ Asbestosis
- ⓓ None of these

Ans. ⓐ

Q-69. Which of the following is not a carrier of vector-borne diseases?

   ⓐ Mosquito   **ⓑ** Bugs

   ⓒ Ticks   **ⓓ** Butterflies

Ans. **ⓓ**

Q-70. The scientific study of climate patterns is called:

   ⓐ Limnology   **ⓑ** Meteorology

   ⓒ Climatology   **ⓓ** Ethology

Ans. **ⓒ**

Q-71. Which of the following is not a type of precipitation?

   ⓐ Rain   **ⓑ** Hail

   ⓒ Snow   **ⓓ** Wind

Ans. **ⓓ**

Q-72. What is the measure of acidity or basicity of an aqueous solution?

   ⓐ pH   **ⓑ** Decibel

   ⓒ Frequency   **ⓓ** Wave length

Ans. **ⓐ**

Q-73. What is the pH of water?

   ⓐ 7   **ⓑ** 8.5

   ⓒ 16   **ⓓ** 1

Ans. **ⓐ**

Q-74. The rate at which temperature drops with the increase in altitude is called:

   ⓐ Global warming

   ⓑ Atmospheric pressure

   ⓒ Environmental Lapse Rate (ELR)

   ⓓ None of these

Ans. **ⓒ**

Q-75. An underground source of water is called:

   ⓐ Stream   **ⓑ** Lake

   ⓒ Aquifer   **ⓓ** Canal

Ans. **ⓒ**

Q-76. Substances that cause cancer in living beings are called:

   ⓐ Pollutants

   ⓑ CFCs

   ⓒ Carcinogens

   ⓓ None of these

Ans. **ⓒ**

Q-77. A legal limit imposed on countries or companies regarding the amount of greenhouse gas emission is called:

   ⓐ Emission cap

   ⓑ Kyoto Protocol

   ⓒ International treaty

   ⓓ None of these

Ans. **ⓐ**

Q-78. A bay at the mouth of a water body in which large quantities of freshwater and seawater mix together is called:

   ⓐ A gulf   **ⓑ** A coral reef

   ⓒ An estuary   **ⓓ** An island

Ans. **ⓒ**

Q-79. The study of genes and hereditary characteristics among humans is called:

   ⓐ Ecology   **ⓒ** Eugenics

   ⓑ Evolution   **ⓓ** None of these

Ans. **ⓒ**

Q-80. The depletion of dissolved oxygen in water is called:

- ⓐ Anorexia
- ⓑ Hypoxia
- ⓒ Hydroxia
- ⓓ None of these

Ans. ⓑ

Q-81. Leukaemia is:

- ⓐ A form of bone marrow cancer
- ⓑ A food disorder
- ⓒ A type of cyclone
- ⓓ None of these

Ans. ⓐ

Q-82. The study of oceans and ocean life is called:

- ⓐ Oceanography
- ⓑ Hydrology
- ⓒ Ecology
- ⓓ Limnology

Ans. ⓐ

Q-83. Fish that live at or near the water surface are called:

- ⓐ Benthos
- ⓑ Pelagic
- ⓒ Demersal
- ⓓ Groundfish

Ans. ⓑ

Q-84. Which of the following is not a radioactive element?

- ⓐ Plutonium
- ⓑ Sodium
- ⓒ Uranium
- ⓓ Radium

Ans. ⓑ

Q-85. Radon is:

- ⓐ A radioactive element
- ⓑ A radioactive gas
- ⓒ A radar system
- ⓓ None of these

Ans. ⓑ

Q-86. A region over which water flows into a river, stream or reservoir is called:

- ⓐ Dam
- ⓑ Tributary
- ⓒ Estuary
- ⓓ Watershed

Ans. ⓓ

Q-87. A group of islands that lie close together is called:

- ⓐ Continent
- ⓑ Archipelago
- ⓒ Bunding
- ⓓ None of these

Ans. ⓑ

Q-88. A stretch of water that has been bypassed by the main flow of a stream but is still connected to it is called a:

- ⓐ Stream
- ⓑ Tributary
- ⓒ Backwater
- ⓓ Bay

Ans. ⓒ

Q-89. When embankments are constructed around crop fields to conserve water and soil, the practice is called:

- ⓐ Soil conservation
- ⓑ Dam building
- ⓒ Watershed management
- ⓓ Bunding

Ans. ⓓ

Q-90. Small marine polyps that occur in colonies found in warm shallow sea water are called:

- ⓐ Coral
- ⓑ Reef
- ⓒ Plankton
- ⓓ None of these

Ans. ⓐ

Q-91. The area drained by a major river or its tributaries is called a/an:

    ⓐ Bay   ⓑ Estuary
    ⓒ Catchment area   ⓓ Embankment

Ans. ⓒ

Q-92. A grained metamorphic rock with a banded structure that is formed during mountain building or volcanic activity is called:

    ⓐ Igneous rock   ⓑ Granite rock
    ⓒ Gneiss   ⓓ None of these

Ans. ⓒ

Q-93. A deep valley with steep and rocky side walls is called a:

    ⓐ Mountain   ⓑ Plateau
    ⓒ Gorge   ⓓ None of these

Ans. ⓒ

Q-94. The dead organic content of the soil which increases its fertility is called:

    ⓐ Humus
    ⓑ Fossils
    ⓒ Terricolous animals
    ⓓ None of these

Ans. ⓐ

Q-95. A piece of land jutting out into the sea is called:

    ⓐ An estuary   ⓑ An island
    ⓒ A bay   ⓓ A peninsula

Ans. ⓓ

Q-96. An area which is reserved for the conservation of animals is called:

    ⓐ Zoo   ⓑ Sanctuary
    ⓒ Forests   ⓓ None of these

Ans. ⓑ

Q-97. The layer of solid rocks at the bottom of the three sub-layers of soil is called:

    ⓐ Sub-soil   ⓑ Top soil
    ⓒ Bedrock   ⓓ None of these

Ans. ⓒ

Q-98. A mass of snow and ice that slowly moves away from its place of formation is called:

    ⓐ Glacier   ⓑ Mountain
    ⓒ Island   ⓓ None of these

Ans. ⓐ

Q-99. An enormous mass of ice that floats on big water bodies, with only a small portion of it visible above the water surface is called:

    ⓐ Glacier   ⓑ Iceberg
    ⓒ Mountain   ⓓ None of these

Ans. ⓑ

Q-100. A mass of land that is surrounded by water on all sides, and is smaller in size than a continent is called:

    ⓐ Gully   ⓑ Island
    ⓒ Bay   ⓓ Gulf

Ans. ⓑ

QUIZ BOOKS

ENGLISH IMPROVEMENT

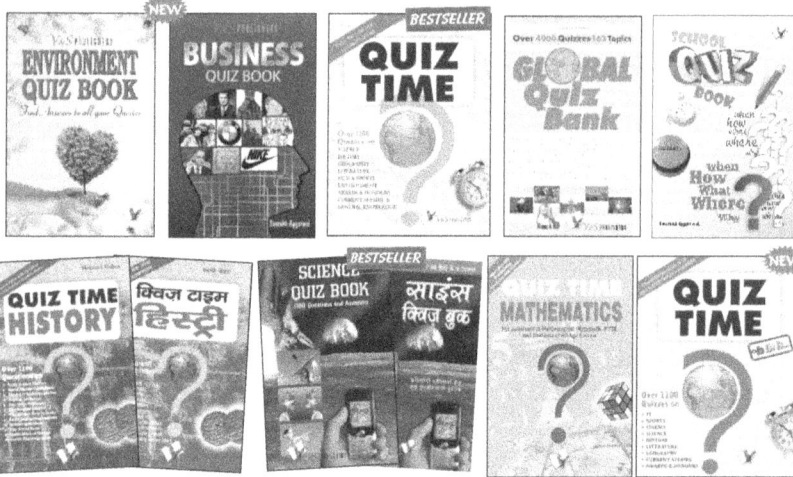

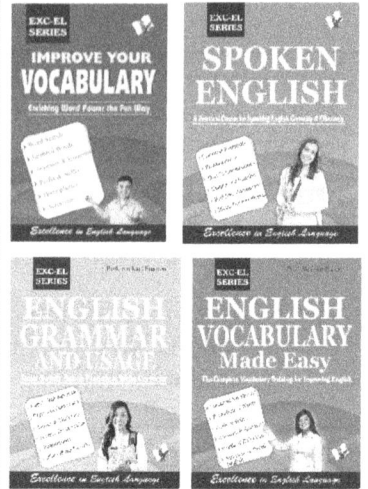

ACTIVITIES BOOK

QUOTES/SAYINGS

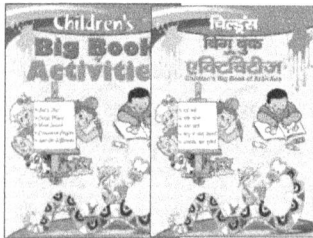

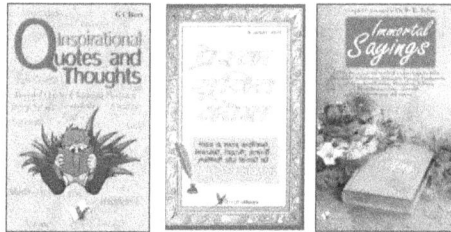

BIOGRAPHIES

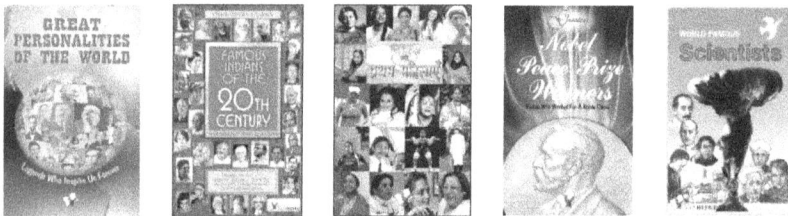

IELTS TECH

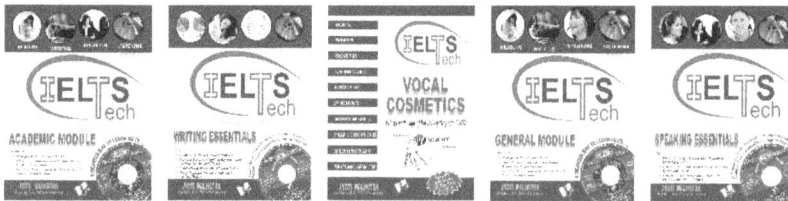

CHILDREN SCIENCE LIBRARY

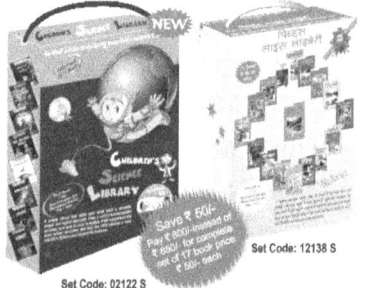

COMPUTER BOOKS

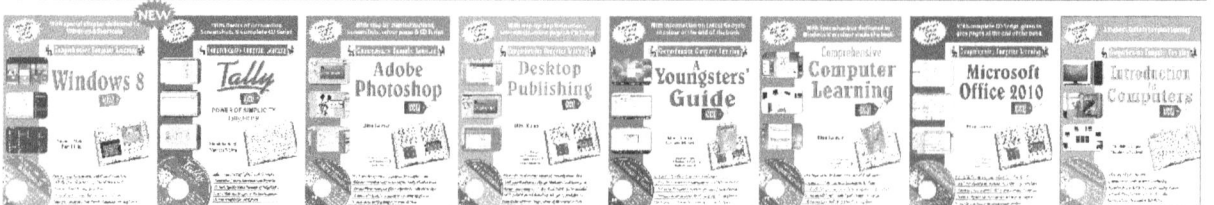

Also available in Hindi

Also available in Hindi